.Atlas of Pediatric Echocardiography

Atlas of Pediatric Echocardiography

Filip Kucera

Consultant Pediatric Cardiologist,
Great Ormond Street Hospital (GOSH),
London,
United Kingdom

ELSEVIER

Elsevier
Radarweg 29, PO Box 211, 1000 AE Amsterdam, Netherlands
The Boulevard, Langford Lane, Kidlington, Oxford OX5 1GB, United Kingdom
50 Hampshire Street, 5th Floor, Cambridge, MA 02139, United States

Notices
Knowledge and best practice in this field are constantly changing. As new research and experience broaden our understanding, changes in research methods, professional practices, or medical treatment may become necessary.

Practitioners and researchers must always rely on their own experience and knowledge in evaluating and using any information, methods, compounds, or experiments described herein. In using such information or methods they should be mindful of their own safety and the safety of others, including parties for whom they have a professional responsibility.

To the fullest extent of the law, neither the Publisher nor the authors, contributors, or editors, assume any liability for any injury and/or damage to persons or property as a matter of products liability, negligence or otherwise, or from any use or operation of any methods, products, instructions, or ideas contained in the material herein.

Library of Congress Cataloging-in-Publication Data
A catalog record for this book is available from the Library of Congress

British Library Cataloguing-in-Publication Data
A catalogue record for this book is available from the British Library

ISBN: 978-0-323-75981-6

For information on all Elsevier publications visit our website at
https://www.elsevier.com/books-and-journals

Publisher: Dolores Meloni
Acquisitions Editor: Sarah Barth
Editorial Project Manager: Billie Jean Fernandez
Production Project Manager: Kiruthika Govindaraju
Cover Designer: Victoria Pearson

Typeset by TNQ Technologies

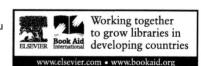

Working together
to grow libraries in
developing countries

www.elsevier.com • www.bookaid.org

To Slavka, my beloved wife,

and

Klara, Sofie, and Dominik, our beloved children,

for their endless love and support.

Contents

About the author.. ix

Foreword... xi

Acknowledgments... xiii

List of abbreviations.. xv

PART A General considerations

CHAPTER 1   Normal transthoracic echocardiogram in a child.... 3

CHAPTER 2   Segmental approach to congenital heart disease ..27

PART B Congenital heart defects

CHAPTER 3   Atrial septal defects..45

CHAPTER 4   Ventricular septal defects 53

CHAPTER 5   Atrio-ventricular septal defects 63

CHAPTER 6   Diseases of the mitral valve 71

CHAPTER 7   Diseases of the tricuspid valve...............................81

CHAPTER 8   Diseases of the left ventricular outflow tract.........89

CHAPTER 9   Diseases of the right ventricular outflow tract..... 101

CHAPTER 10   Double outlet right ventricle...................................111

CHAPTER 11   Tetralogy of Fallot 121

CHAPTER 12   Transposition of the great arteries...................... 133

CHAPTER 13   Congenitally corrected transposition of the
great arteries... 141

CHAPTER 14   Persistent truncus arteriosus............................. 147

CHAPTER 15   Functionally single ventricle 155

CHAPTER 16   Patent ductus arteriosus and aorto-pulmonary
window... 173

CHAPTER 17   Coarctation of the aorta and interrupted
aortic arch.. 181

CHAPTER 18   Vascular rings 191

CHAPTER 19 Pulmonary and systemic venous anomalies......... 199

CHAPTER 20 Congenital coronary artery abnormalities............ 211

PART C Acquired heart diseases and other conditions

CHAPTER 21 Myocarditis 221

CHAPTER 22 Cardiomyopathies 225

CHAPTER 23 Kawasaki disease 237

CHAPTER 24 Rheumatic fever.. 241

CHAPTER 25 Infective endocarditis 247

CHAPTER 26 Pericardial disease... 253

CHAPTER 27 Cardiac tumors 263

CHAPTER 28 Pulmonary hypertension..................................... 269

CHAPTER 29 Common genetic disorders associated with heart disease... 275

CHAPTER 30 Mechanical circulatory support and heart transplantation.. 283

Index...291

About the author

Dr. Filip Kucera is a consultant pediatric cardiologist at Great Ormond Street Hospital (GOSH) in London, one of the world's leading centers for pediatric cardiology and cardiac surgery. Due to high volumes of patients, he has vast experience in echocardiography of congenital and acquired heart disease in children. He was an invited speaker at several international conferences, giving talks on echocardiography. He also published a number of articles in medical journals and was part of several grant applications. He has regularly been involved in courses on pediatric echocardiography at GOSH. The idea to write "The Atlas of Pediatric Echocardiography" arose from his enthusiasm and experience of teaching echocardiography across various pediatric subspecialties.

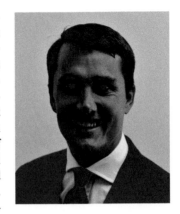

Foreword

This book provides high-quality echocardiographic images produced by Filip Kucera over his years of training and clinical practice at Great Ormond Street Hospital (GOSH). Although the author of this book may not be recognized by the World experts in pediatric echocardiography, many of them may be positively surprised by the wonderful piece of work he has created for this publication. It is however no surprise to me as I have known Filip from his (and mine) native Prague and since his arrival to GOSH. Filip's excellent and well-organized work has culminated in this outstanding atlas demonstrating illustrative images of the heart conditions commonly seen during childhood.

The aim of this book is not to teach echocardiography or the morphology of cardiac abnormalities in detail but rather to offer a simple way to establish correct, mainly preoperative, diagnosis and how to define abnormalities by linking "*Andersonian*" terminology of congenital cardiac lesions with illustrative echocardiographic images. The first chapter focuses on practical scanning of children and the projections used to obtain a correct, high-quality image of each cardiac structure and an introduction to sequential segmental approach for assessment of congenital heart abnormalities. All chapters on individual heart abnormalities are structured similarly: introduction, definition, brief clinical description, and treatment. Short, concise, and conclusive. Filip has then demonstrated a large collection of representative images with a short description on how to produce the image and comments on hemodynamic assessment where relevant. There is a section on echocardiographic imaging of acquired heart conditions that include a collection of images of diseases commonly seen by pediatric cardiologists, from myocarditis and cardiomyopathy through to cardiac infection and tumors. In some chapters, such as "*Mechanical circulatory support and heart transplantation*," Filip has shared his experiences working with the heart failure team at GOSH.

As one of the experts in pediatric and prenatal echocardiography and one of the examiners for the European Accreditation in Echocardiography of Congenital Heart Disease under the European Association of Cardiovascular Imaging (EACVI), I believe this book will serve as an introduction for examination preparation by learning the fundamental practical approach to echocardiographic imaging of heart conditions in children and young adults. The colleagues that will benefit from reading this book are those eager to improve their pediatric congenital echocardiography technique and colleagues considering practicing pediatric cardiology as an additional subspecialty to pediatrics or neonatology. Enjoy reading!

Professor Jan Marek, MD, PhD, FESC
Clinical Lead for Echocardiography
Professor of Cardiology
Great Ormond Street Hospital for Children
and Institute of Cardiovascular Sciences
University College London, United Kingdom

Acknowledgments

My special thanks and appreciation is extended to those who have provided invaluable advice in writing the first edition of this book. In particular, I would like to thank Professor Jan Marek who is the Clinical Lead for Echocardiography at Great Ormond Street Hospital. I am very much indebted to him for having reviewed the content of the book, but also for allowing me to use some of his pictures, without which the book would not be complete. Jan has been an incredible teacher, mentor, and inspiration to me, always willing to share his knowledge and experience. It is a great honor that the foreword to this book was written by such a world expert.

I am also very grateful to Emma Carter, the Lead Cardiac Physiologist at Great Ormond Street Hospital, for her extensive review of the book. Her review was key in the editorial process of this book and helped to ensure the text was precise and comprehensible.

I would also like to acknowledge Dr. Oliver Tann who is the Clinical Lead for Cardiac CT and MRI at Great Ormond Street Hospital. Oliver has provided me with some stunning CT pictures, which I used to better illustrate the anatomy of various types of vascular rings. I am very thankful for his permission to use them in my book.

Special thanks go to Klara, Sofie, and Dominik for being the photography models in this book.

Finally, I would like to thank all my consultant colleagues from Great Ormond Street Hospital and the Children's Heart Centre in Prague. They helped to shape my career and have influenced who I am today. It is only thanks to them that I was able to write this book. All the pictures in this book are from cardiac patients at Great Ormond Street Hospital, and therefore one last thanks goes to them.

List of abbreviations

aLAo	atretic left aortic arch
alPM	anterolateral papillary muscle
ALSCA	aberrant left subclavian artery
aMV	anterior mitral valve leaflet
ANT. LIMB	anterior limb of TSM
Ao	aorta
Ao D	aortic diverticulum
AoV	aortic valve
ARSCA	aberrant right subclavian artery
aRV	atrialized right ventricle
Asc. Ao	ascending aorta
ASD	atrial septal defect
aTV	antero-superior leaflet of the tricuspid valve
AV	atrio-ventricular
BCT	brachiocephalic trunk
cAVV	common AV valve
CCV	common collector vein
CND	conduit
COE T	coeliac trunk
CONF	confluence of pulmonary veins
CS	coronary sinus
CVL	central venous line
DAo	descending aorta
DIAPH	diaphragm
EUST V	Eustachian valve
fRV	functional right ventricle
HMGR	homograft
HV	hepatic vein
IAS	interatrial septum
ICD	implantable cardioverter defibrillator
INF	sinus venosus inferior defect
IS	infundibular septum
iTV	inferior leaflet of the tricuspid valve
IVC	inferior vena cava
IVS	interventricular septum
Komm D	Kommerell's diverticulum
L Ao	left aortic arch
L-PDA	left ductus/ligamentum arteriosum
LA	left atrium
LAD	left anterior descending coronary artery
LAVV	left atrio-ventricular valve
LCC	left coronary cusp
LCCA	left common carotid artery
LCx	left circumflex coronary artery

LIV	left innominate vein
LLPV	left lower pulmonary vein
LMB	left main bronchus
LMCA	left main coronary artery
LPA	left pulmonary artery
LSCA	left subclavian artery
LSVC	left superior vena cava
LUPV	left upper pulmonary vein
LV	left ventricle
LV AW	left ventricular anterior wall
LV IW	left ventricular inferior wall
LVd	*LV* end-diastolic diamete*r*
LVs	*LV* end-systolic diameter
mBT	modified Blalock-Taussig shunt
mLV	morphological left ventricle
mRV	morphological right ventricle
MV	mitral valve
MVR	prosthetic mitral valve
NCC	noncoronary cusp
O	esophagus
PA	pulmonary artery
PAV	pulmonary valve
PE	pericardial effusion
PERIC	pericardium
pmPM	posteromedial papillary muscle
pMV	posterior mitral valve leaflet
POST. LIMB	posterior limb TSM
PR	pulmonary regurgitation
PRIM	ostium primum ASD
PW	left ventricular posterior wall
R Ao	right aortic arch
RA	right atrium
RAVV	right atrio-ventricular valve
RCA	right coronary artery
RCC	right coronary cusp
RCCA	right common carotid artery
rCH	rudimentary chamber
RIV	right innominate vein
RLPV	right lower pulmonary vein
RMB	right main bronchus
RPA	right pulmonary artery
RSCA	right subclavian artery
RSVC	right superior vena cava
RUPV	right upper pulmonary vein
RV	right ventricle
RV FW	right ventricular free wall
SEC	ostium secundum atrial septal defect
SMA	superior mesenteric artery

STJ	sinotubular junction
sTV	septal tricuspid valve leaflet
SUP	sinus venosus superior defect
SV	single ventricle
T	trachea
TR	tricuspid regurgitation
TRU	truncus
TSM	septomarginal trabecula
TV	tricuspid valve
VSD	ventricular septal defect
VV	vertical vein (TAPVC)

General considerations

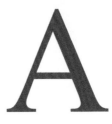

Normal transthoracic echocardiogram in a child

Transthoracic echocardiography is the first-line imaging modality for the diagnosis of congenital and acquired heart conditions in children. It allows a detailed morphological and functional examination of different cardiac structures. A standard echocardiographic study consists of two-dimensional (2D) imaging, motion mode (M-mode), and Doppler imaging.

The analysis of cardiac anatomy is based on cross-sectional visualization of the heart in conventional 2D planes, which show the real-time movement of cardiac structures. Standard views include subcostal, apical, parasternal, and suprasternal views. M-mode echocardiography is a one-dimensional imaging technique that records the real-time movement of cardiac structures over multiple cardiac cycles.

Doppler imaging comprises color flow and spectral Doppler modalities. Color flow mapping (CFM) is a 2D representation of the direction and velocity of blood flow within a predefined sector that is superimposed on the 2D image. By definition, flow toward the probe is red and flow away from the probe is blue. Depending on the selected Nyquist limit, lighter color shades show higher flow velocities. Spectral Doppler is a record of blood flow velocity over time. It is further divided into pulsed-wave Doppler used for low blood flow velocities, and continuous-wave Doppler for high blood flow velocities.

Two-dimensional echocardiography, color flow Doppler

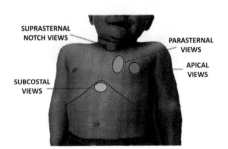

SUPRASTERNAL NOTCH VIEWS

PARASTERNAL VIEWS

APICAL VIEWS

SUBCOSTAL VIEWS

FIGURE 1

Location of different echocardiographic windows. Subcostal window (yellow), apical window (green), parasternal window (blue), suprasternal window (red).

Atlas of Pediatric Echocardiography. https://doi.org/10.1016/B978-0-323-75981-6.00029-7

Subcostal views

A standard echocardiographic study begins with subcostal views. The probe is placed on the upper abdomen, just below the lower edge of the sternum. Images of the cardiac and vascular structures are acquired through the liver. In very small children, it is possible to perform the entire echocardiogram from subcostal approach.

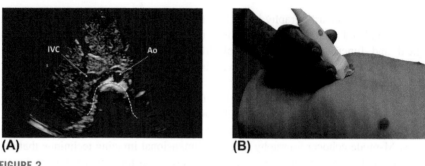

FIGURE 2

(A) Subcostal "situs" view (transverse plane). In normal abdominal situs, the abdominal aorta is to the left and the inferior vena cava to the right of the spine. (B) The probe marker is at the 3 o'clock position. *Ao*, aorta; *IVC*, inferior vena cava.

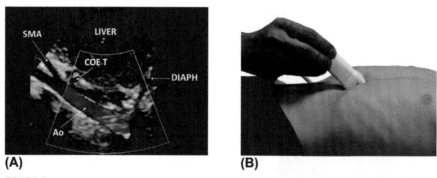

FIGURE 3

(A) Color flow Doppler of the abdominal aorta from the subcostal view. Pulsed-wave Doppler interrogation of the abdominal aorta is performed from this view. (B) The probe is at the 6 o'clock position, angulated inferiorly. *Ao*, aorta; *COE T*, celiac trunk; *DIAPH*, diaphragm; *SMA*, superior mesenteric artery.

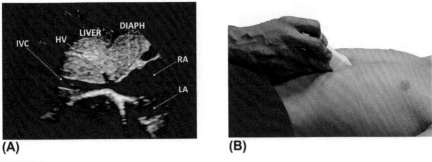

FIGURE 4

(A) Subcostal view showing the drainage of the inferior vena cava and the hepatic veins into the right atrium. (B) The probe at the 6 o'clock position, tilted inferiorly and slightly to the patient's left. *DIAPH*, diaphragm; *HV*, hepatic vein; *IVC*, inferior vena cava; *LA*, left atrium; *RA*, right atrium.

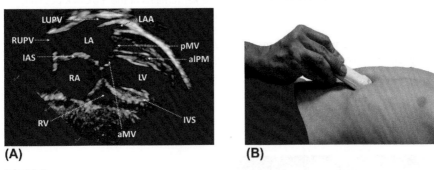

FIGURE 5

(A) Subcostal long-axis (four-chamber) view. The cardiac chambers, atrial and ventricular septae, and upper pulmonary veins are visualized. (B) The probe is at the 3 o'clock position, angulated inferiorly. *aIPM*, anterolateral papillary muscle; *aMV*, anterior mitral valve leaflet; *IAS*, interatrial septum; *IVS*, interventricular septum; *LA*, left atrium; *LAA*, left atrial appendage; *LUPV*, left upper pulmonary vein; *LV*, left ventricle; *pMV*, posterior mitral valve leaflet; *RA*, right atrium; *RUPV*, right upper pulmonary vein; *RV*, right ventricle.

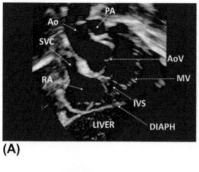

(A)

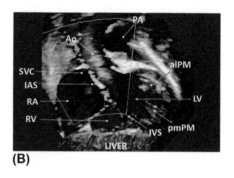

(B)

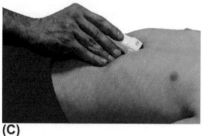

(C)

FIGURE 6

(A) Subcostal long-axis view showing the entire left ventricular outflow tract with the proximal ascending aorta. (B) Corresponding color flow Doppler. (C) The probe is further angulated inferiorly as compared to the previous figure. The marker remains at the 3 o'clock position. *alPM*, anterolateral papillary muscle; *Ao*, aorta; *DIAPH*, diaphragm; *IAS*, interatrial septum; *IVS*, interventricular septum; *LV*, left ventricle; *MV*, mitral valve; *PA*, pulmonary artery; *pmPM*, posteromedial papillary muscle; *RA*, right atrium; *RV*, right ventricle; *SVC*, superior vena cava.

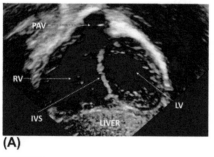

(A)

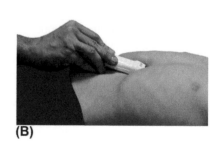

(B)

FIGURE 7

(A) Subcostal long-axis view showing both ventricles and the right ventricular outflow tract. (B) This view is obtained by a maximal inferior angulation of the probe. The marker is at the 3 o'clock position. *alPM*, anterolateral papillary muscle; *IVS*, interventricular septum; *LV*, left ventricle; *PA*, pulmonary artery; *PAV*, pulmonary valve; *pmPM*, posteromedial papillary muscle; *RV*, right ventricle.

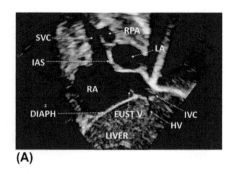
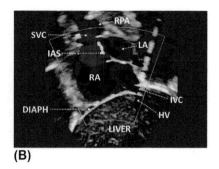

(A)   **(B)**

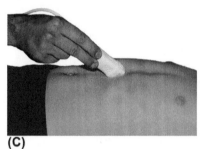

(C)

FIGURE 8

(A) Subcostal short-axis (bicaval) view showing both caval veins and atria. (B) Flow across the superior and inferior caval veins. (C) The probe is at the 5 o'clock position, tilted slightly to the patient's left. *DIAPH*, diaphragm; *EUST V*, Eustachian valve; *HV*, hepatic vein; *IAS*, interatrial septum; *IVC*, inferior vena cava; *LA*, left atrium; *RA*, right atrium; *RPA*, right pulmonary artery; *SVC*, superior vena cava.

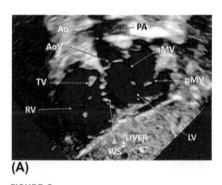
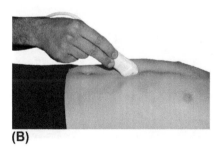

(A)   **(B)**

FIGURE 9

(A) Subcostal short-axis view showing the left ventricular outflow tract and the mitral valve. The interventricular septum is visualized en face. (B) The probe is slightly tilted to the patient's right as compared to the previous figure. *aMV*, anterior mitral valve leaflet; *Ao*, aorta; *AoV*, aortic valve; *IVS*, interventricular septum; *LV*, left ventricle; *PA*, pulmonary artery; *pMV*, posterior mitral valve leaflet; *RV*, right ventricle; *TV*, tricuspid valve.

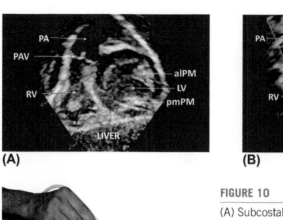

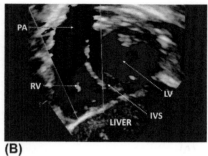

(A)   **(B)**

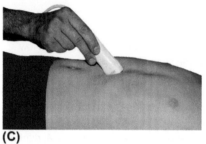

(C)

FIGURE 10

(A) Subcostal short-axis view showing the entire right ventricular outflow tract. (B) Corresponding color flow Doppler. (C) The probe is further tilted to the patient's right as compared to the previous figure. *aIPM*, anterolateral papillary muscle; *IVS*, interventricular septum; *LV*, left ventricle; *PA*, pulmonary artery; *PAV*, pulmonary valve; *pmPM*, posteromedial papillary muscle; *RV*, right ventricle.

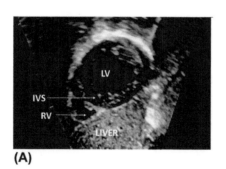

(A)

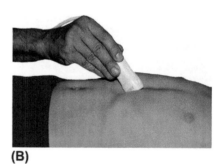

(B)

FIGURE 11

(A) Subcostal short-axis view with cross-sectional view of both ventricles. (B) The probe is further tilted to the patient's right as compared to the previous figure. *IVS*, interventricular septum; *LV*, left ventricle; *RV*, right ventricle.

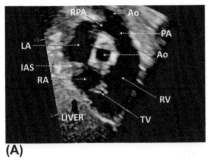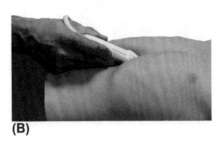

(A)   **(B)**

FIGURE 12

(A) Subcostal short-axis view demonstrating both atria, the tricuspid valve, and the entire right ventricular outflow tract. (B) This view is obtained by rotating the probe marker to the 1 o'clock position. The probe is slightly tilted to the patient's left. *Ao*, aorta; *IAS*, interatrial septum; *LA*, left atrium; *LPA*, left pulmonary artery; *PA*, pulmonary artery; *RA*, right atrium; *RPA*, right pulmonary artery; *RV*, right ventricle; *TV*, tricuspid valve.

Apical views

In apical views, cardiac structures are visualized with the probe positioned over the apex of the heart. The imaging quality can be improved, especially in older children, by placing the patient into a left lateral decubitus position with the left arm placed under the head. This causes the heart to move closer to the chest wall, away from the left lung. In smaller children, apical windows are usually medial to the left nipple, while in older children they are located more laterally.

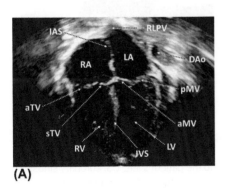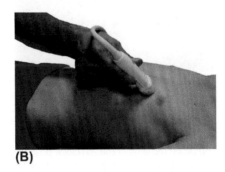

(A)   **(B)**

FIGURE 13

(A) Apical four-chamber view showing both atria, ventricles and atrio-ventricular valves. (B) The probe is at the 2 o'clock position, tilted to the patient's left. *aMV*, anterior mitral valve leaflet; *aTV*, antero-superior tricuspid valve leaflet; *DAo*, descending aorta; *IAS*, interatrial septum; *IVS*, interventricular septum; *LA*, left atrium; *LV*, left ventricle; *pMV*, posterior mitral valve leaflet; *RA*, right atrium; *RLPV*, right lower pulmonary vein; *RV*, right ventricle; *sTV*, septal tricuspid valve leaflet.

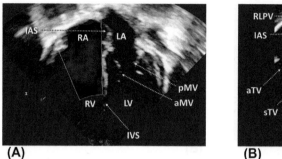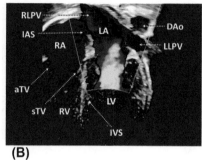

(A)   **(B)**

FIGURE 14

Apical four-chamber view. (A) Color flow Doppler of the tricuspid inflow. (B) Drainage of the right and left lower pulmonary veins into the left atrium and the transmitral inflow. *aMV*, anterior mitral valve leaflet; *aTV*, antero-superior tricuspid valve leaflet; *DAo*, descending aorta; *IAS*, interatrial septum; *IVS*, interventricular septum; *LA*, left atrium; *LLPV*, left lower pulmonary vein; *LV*, left ventricle; *pMV*, posterior mitral valve leaflet; *RA*, right atrium; *RLPV*, right lower pulmonary vein; *RV*, right ventricle; *sTV*, septal tricuspid valve leaflet.

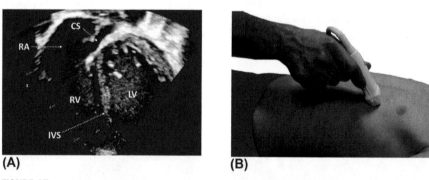

(A)   **(B)**

FIGURE 15

(A) Visualization of the coronary sinus from the apical view. (B) This view is obtained by a superior angulation of the probe as compared to the standard apical four-chamber view. The probe remains at the 2 o'clock position, tilted to the patient's left. *CS*, coronary sinus; *IVS*, interventricular septum; *LV*, left ventricle; *RA*, right atrium; *RV*, right ventricle.

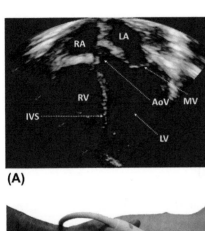

(A)

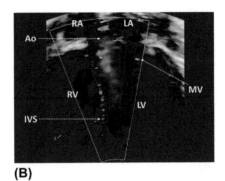

(B)

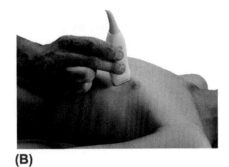

(C)

FIGURE 16

(A) Apical five-chamber view showing the subvalvar and valvar component of the left ventricular outflow tract. (B) Corresponding color flow Doppler. (C) This view is obtained by an inferior angulation of the probe as compared to the standard apical four-chamber view. The probe is at the 2 o'clock position, tilted to the patient's left. *AoV*, aortic valve; *IVS*, interventricular septum; *LA*, left atrium; *LV*, left ventricle; *MV*, mitral valve; *RA*, right atrium; *RV*, right ventricle.

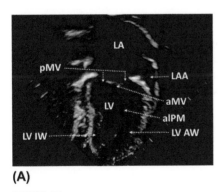

(A)

(B)

FIGURE 17

(A) Apical two-chamber view demonstrating the left atrium, the left atrial appendage and the left ventricle. (B) This view is obtained from the apical four-chamber view by counter clockwise rotation of the probe marker to the 10 o'clock position. *alPM*, anterolateral papillary muscle; *aMV*, anterior mitral valve leaflet; *LA*, left atrium; *LAA*, left atrial appendage; *LV AW*, left ventricular anterior wall; *LV IW*, left ventricular inferior wall; *LV*, left ventricle; *pMV*, posterior mitral valve leaflet.

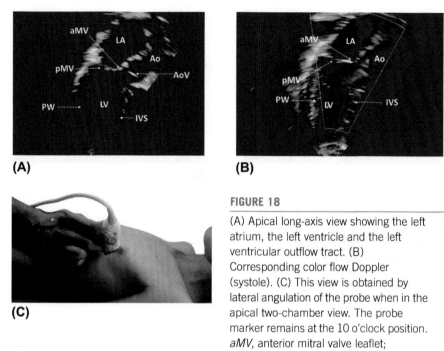

(A)

(B)

(C)

FIGURE 18

(A) Apical long-axis view showing the left atrium, the left ventricle and the left ventricular outflow tract. (B) Corresponding color flow Doppler (systole). (C) This view is obtained by lateral angulation of the probe when in the apical two-chamber view. The probe marker remains at the 10 o'clock position. *aMV*, anterior mitral valve leaflet; *Ao*, aorta; *AoV*, aortic valve; *IVS*, interventricular septum; *LA*, left atrium; *LV*, left ventricle; *pMV*, posterior mitral valve leaflet; *PW*, left ventricular posterior wall.

Parasternal views

Parasternal views include the parasternal long-axis and short-axis views. The probe is to the left of the sternum, close to the level of the fourth intercostal space. In the parasternal long-axis view, the probe marker points to the right shoulder, while in parasternal short-axis view, it is directed toward the left shoulder. Both views are perpendicular to each other.

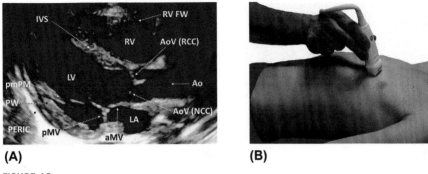

(A)   **(B)**

FIGURE 19

(A) Standard parasternal long-axis view showing the left atrium, the left ventricle and the left ventricular outflow tract. M-mode measurements of the left ventricular dimensions and function are performed in this view. (B) The probe marker is at the 11 o'clock position (pointing to the patient's right shoulder). *aMV*, anterior mitral valve leaflet; *Ao*, aorta; *AoV (NCC)*, noncoronary cusp of the aortic valve; *AoV (RCC)*, right coronary cusp of the aortic valve; *IVS*, interventricular septum; *LA*, left atrium; *LV*, left ventricle; *PERIC*, pericardium; *pmPM*, posteromedial papillary muscle; *pMV*, posterior mitral valve leaflet; *PW*, left ventricular posterior wall; *RV FW*, right ventricular free wall; *RV*, right ventricle.

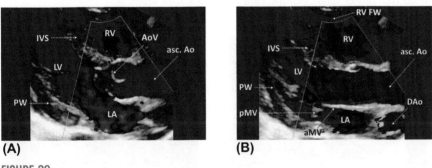

(A)   **(B)**

FIGURE 20

Color flow Doppler from the parasternal long-axis view. (A) Transmitral flow (diastole). (B) Flow across the left ventricular outflow tract (systole). *aMV*, anterior mitral valve leaflet; *asc Ao*, ascending aorta; *AoV*, aortic valve; *DAo*, descending aorta; *IVS*, interventricular septum; *LA*, left atrium; *LV*, left ventricle; *pMV*, posterior mitral valve leaflet; *PW*, left ventricular posterior wall; *RV FW*, right ventricular free wall; *RV*, right ventricle.

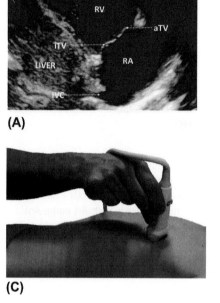

(A)

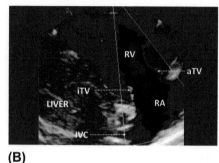

(B)

FIGURE 21

(A) Parasternal long-axis view showing the right atrium, the right ventricle, and the tricuspid valve. (B) Flow across the tricuspid valve as demonstrated on color flow Doppler. (C) This view is obtained by angulation of the probe to the patient's left when in the standard parasternal long-axis view. The probe marker is at an 11 o'clock position. *aTV*, antero-superior tricuspid valve leaflet; *iTV*, inferior tricuspid valve leaflet; *IVC*, inferior vena cava; *RA*, right atrium; *RV*, right ventricle.

(C)

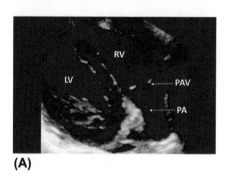

(A)

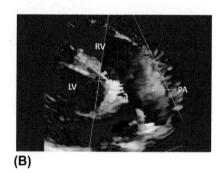

(B)

FIGURE 22

(A) Parasternal long-axis view showing the entire right ventricular outflow tract. (B) Blood flow across the right ventricular outflow tract as demonstrated on color flow Doppler. (C) This view is obtained from the standard parasternal long-axis view by angulation of the probe to the patient's right. The probe marker remains at the 11 o'clock position. *LV*, left ventricle; *PA*, pulmonary artery; *PAV*, pulmonary valve; *RV*, right ventricle.

(C)

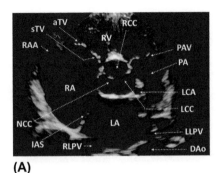 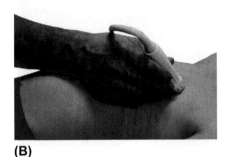

(A)   **(B)**

FIGURE 23

(A) Standard parasternal short-axis view showing both atria, the tricuspid valve and the entire right ventricular outflow tract. En face view of the aortic valve. (B) The probe is at the 2 o'clock position (pointing to the left shoulder) and tilted to the patient's left. *AoV*, aortic valve; *aTV*, antero-superior tricuspid valve leaflet; *DAo*, descending aorta; *IAS*, interatrial septum; *LA*, left atrium; *LCA*, left coronary artery; *LCC*, left coronary cusp; *LLPV*, left lower pulmonary vein; *LUPV*, left upper pulmonary vein; *NCC*, non-coronary cusp of the aortic valve; *PA*, pulmonary artery; *PAV*, pulmonary valve; *RA*, right atrium; *RAA*, right atrial appendage; *RCC*, right coronary cusp; *RLPV*, right lower pulmonary vein; *RV*, right ventricle; *sTV*, septal tricuspid leaflet.

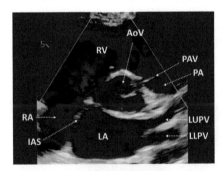

FIGURE 24

Tricuspid inflow as demonstrated on color flow Doppler. *AoV*, aortic valve; *LA*, left atrium; *LLPV*, left lower pulmonary vein; *LUPV*, left upper pulmonary vein; *PA*, pulmonary artery; *PAV*, pulmonary valve; *RA*, right atrium; *RV*, right ventricle.

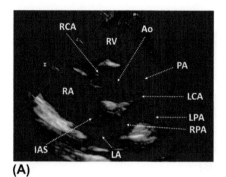 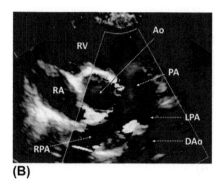

(A)   **(B)**

FIGURE 25

(A) Parasternal short-axis view obtained by a slight inferior tilt of the probe (ultrasound beam directed upwards). This view demonstrates the bifurcation of the pulmonary artery. (B) Corresponding color flow Doppler showing flow in both branch pulmonary arteries. *Ao*, aorta; *DAo*, descending aorta; *LCA*, left coronary artery; *LPA*, left pulmonary artery; *LV*, left ventricle; *PA*, pulmonary artery; *RA*, right atrium; *RCA*, right coronary artery; *RPA*, right pulmonary artery; *RV*, right ventricle.

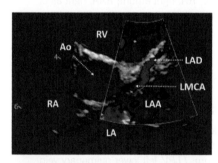

FIGURE 26

Color flow Doppler obtained from a zoomed parasternal short-axis view, illustrating flow in the left coronary artery. *Ao*, aorta; *LA*, left atrium; *LAA*, left atrial appendage; *LAD*, left anterior descending coronary artery; *LMCA*, left main coronary artery; *RA*, right atrium; *RV*, right ventricle.

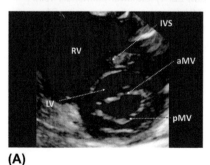 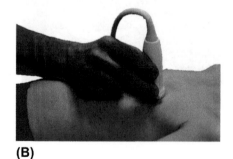

(A)   **(B)**

FIGURE 27

(A) Parasternal short-axis view of the mitral valve. There is a view of the valve en face and the interventricular septum. (B) This view is obtained by a slight medial tilt of the probe or by a slight movement of the probe in a latero-caudal direction. The probe marker remains at the 2 o'clock position. *aMV*, anterior mitral valve leaflet; *IVS*, interventricular septum; *LV*, left ventricle; *pMV*, posterior mitral valve leaflet; *RV*, right ventricle.

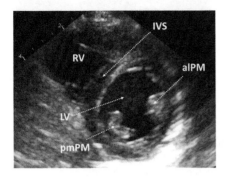

FIGURE 28

Parasternal short-axis view at the level of the papillary muscles of the mitral valve. En face view of both the anterolateral and the posteromedial papillary muscles. Compared to the previous figure, this view is obtained by a further medial tilt of the probe or by a slight movement toward the apex of the heart (in a latero-caudal direction). *alPM*, anterolateral papillary muscle; *IVS*, interventricular septum; *LV*, left ventricle; *pmPM*, posteromedial papillary muscle; *RV*, right ventricle.

Suprasternal notch views

Suprasternal views are obtained by placing the probe over the jugular notch. In particular, they are used to visualize the aortic arch and its branches, the pulmonary artery branches, the head and neck systemic venous system, and the pulmonary veins. The imaging quality is enhanced by the extension of the patient's neck with the chin facing upwards. However, this position is not always well tolerated in small children, sideways rotation of the head and neck may suffice.

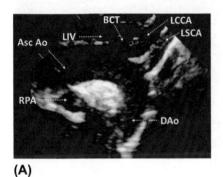

(A)

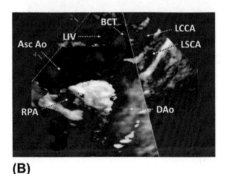

(B)

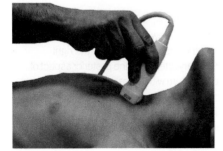

(C)

FIGURE 29

(A) Suprasternal long-axis notch view showing the entire aortic arch, the branches, and part of the descending aorta. (B) Color flow Doppler demonstrating flow in the aorta. (C) The probe is at the 1–2 o'clock position, tilted superiorly. *Asc Ao*, ascending aorta; *BCT*, brachiocephalic trunk; *DAo*, descending aorta; *LCCA*, left common carotid artery; *LIV*, left innominate vein; *LSCA*, left subclavian artery; *RPA*, right pulmonary artery.

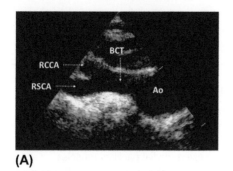

(A)

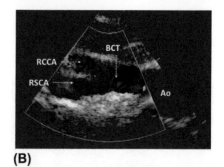

(B)

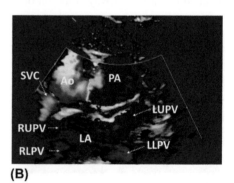

(C)

FIGURE 30

(A) The sidedness of the aortic arch is determined by which side the first aortic branch courses. In a left aortic arch, the brachiocephalic trunk bifurcates to the right. In a right aortic arch, the brachiocephalic trunk courses to the left. (B) Corresponding color flow Doppler. (C) The probe marker is rotated to the 10 o'clock position. *Ao*, aorta; *BCT*, brachiocephalic trunk; *RCCA*, right common carotid artery; *RSCA*, right subclavian artery.

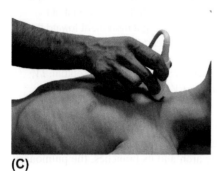

(A)

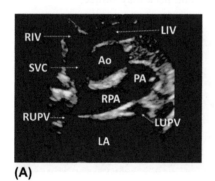

(B)

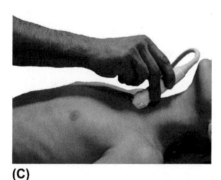

(C)

FIGURE 31

(A) Suprasternal short-axis view (frontal plane). This view shows both innominate veins, the superior vena cava, the right pulmonary artery, and the posterior aspect of the left atrium with the ostia of the pulmonary veins. (B) The drainage of all pulmonary veins into the left atrium ("crab view") demonstrated on color flow Doppler. (C) The probe marker is at the 3 o'clock position. *Ao*, aorta; *LA*, left atrium; *LIV*, left innominate vein; *LLPV*, left lower pulmonary vein; *LUPV*, left upper pulmonary vein; *PA*, pulmonary artery; *RIV*, right innominate vein; *RLPV*, right lower pulmonary vein; *RPA*, right pulmonary artery; *RUPV*, right upper pulmonary vein; *SVC*, superior vena cava.

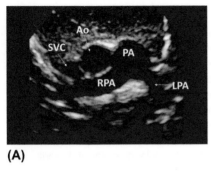

(A)

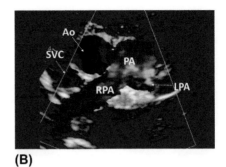

(B)

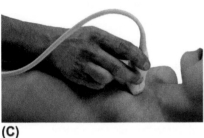

(C)

FIGURE 32

(A) Left subclavicular view ("three vessel view") showing the pulmonary artery, pulmonary artery branches, ascending aorta, and the superior vena cava. (B) Corresponding color flow Doppler. (C) This view is obtained by moving the probe away from the suprasternal notch to just below the left clavicle. The probe is tilted laterally, the marker is at the 2 o'clock position. *Ao*, aorta; *LPA*, left pulmonary artery; *PA*, pulmonary artery; *RPA*, right pulmonary artery; *SVC*, superior vena cava.

Two-dimensional measurements

The figures show how some of the commonly used two-dimensional echocardiographic parameters are measured. Normal pediatric reference ranges are weight and height dependent. A complete list of body surface area indexed values can easily be accessed on the internet via a number of online Z-score calculators.

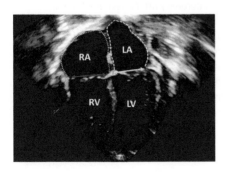

FIGURE 33

Apical four-chamber view. *Orange double arrow* indicates the tricuspid annular diameter, *yellow double arrow* the mitral annular diameter, *dashed line* the left atrial surface area, *dotted line* the right atrial surface area. *LA*, left atrium; *LV*, left ventricle; *RA*, right atrium; *RV*, right ventricle.

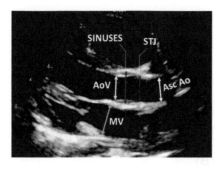

Aortic root measurements from the parasternal long-axis view. *Yellow double arrow* indicates the aortic annular diameter, *blue double arrow* the sinuses of Valsalva diameter, *red double arrow* the sinotubular junction diameter, and *white double arrow* the ascending aorta diameter. *Green double arrow* represents the mitral annular diameter. *AoV*, aortic valve; *asc Ao*, ascending aorta; *MV*, mitral valve; *STJ*, sinotubular junction.

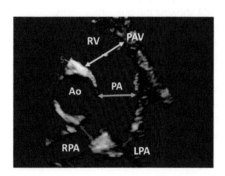

FIGURE 35

Zoomed parasternal short-axis view. *Yellow double arrow* indicates the pulmonary annular diameter, *green double arrow* the pulmonary artery diameter, *orange double arrow* the proximal right pulmonary artery diameter, and the *red double arrow* the left proximal left pulmonary artery diameter. *Ao*, aorta; *LPA*, left pulmonary artery; *PA,* pulmonary artery; *PAV*, pulmonary valve; *RPA*, right pulmonary artery; *RV*, right ventricle.

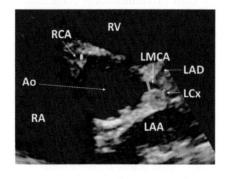

FIGURE 36

Zoomed parasternal short-axis view showing measurements of the proximal coronary arteries. *Yellow line* indicates the right coronary artery, *green line* the left main coronary artery, *red line* the left anterior descending coronary artery, *blue line* the left circumflex coronary artery. *Ao*, aorta; *LAA*, left atrial appendage; *LAD*, left anterior descending coronary artery; *LCx*, left circumflex coronary artery; *LMCA*, left main coronary artery; *RA*, right atrium; *RCA*, right coronary artery; *RV*, right ventricle.

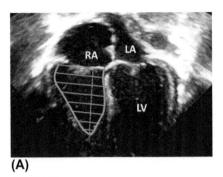 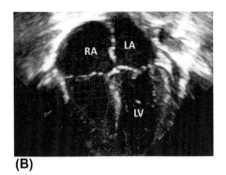

(A)   **(B)**

FIGURE 37

Assessment of right ventricular (RV) systolic function using the right ventricular fractional area change (RV FAC). The RV cavity is traced in an RV-focused apical four-chamber view in both (A) end-diastole and (B) end-systole. The tracings include the papillary muscles and trabeculations. RV FAC is calculated automatically using the formula below and is normal if > 35%.

RV FAC = [(RV end-diastolic area) − (RV end-systolic area)]/(RV end-diastolic area) × 100 [%]

LA, left atrium; *LV*, left ventricle; *RA*, right atrium.

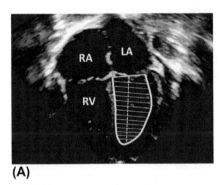 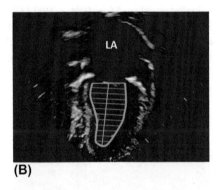

(A)   **(B)**

FIGURE 38

Biplane (Simpson's) method for the evaluation of the left ventricular (LV) ejection fraction (EF). The LV cavity is traced in (A) the apical four-chamber and (B) the apical two-chamber views in both end-systole and end-diastole (end-systolic tracings are not shown in this figure). Automatic calculation of end-systolic and end-diastolic LV volumes allows to determine the EF according to the following equation: **EF = (EDV − ESV) / EDV × 100 [%]** (normal if > 55). *EDV*, end-diastolic volume; *ESV*, end-systolic volume; *LA*, left atrium; *RA*, right atrium; *RV*, right ventricle.

M-mode

The motion mode (M-mode) is a one-dimensional imaging modality that records the real-time movement of cardiac structures along a preselected ultrasound line. M-mode is commonly used for evaluation of the left ventricular dimensions and systolic function, the assessment of right ventricular longitudinal systolic function, and the estimation of inferior vena cava collapsibility, reflecting the right atrial pressure.

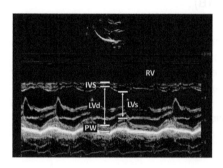

FIGURE 39

Parasternal long-axis M-mode displaying left ventricular dimensions over time. The M-mode cursor is aligned with the tip of the mitral valve leaflets and is perpendicular to the posterior wall of the left ventricle (LV). Besides the measurement of the septal and posterior wall dimensions, this method allows real-time assessment of the LV internal dimensions. The knowledge of the LV end-diastolic diameter (LVd) and the LV end-systolic diameter (LVs) forms the basis for the calculation of shortening fraction (SF) according to the following equation: **SF = (LVd − LVs) / LVd × 100 [%]** (normal if > 25%) Despite numerous limitations, this parameter reflects the LV global systolic function. A simple, approximate way for obtaining ejection fraction (EF) from SF is to multiply the value of SF (in %) by two. More accurately, EF is derived from SF using the Teichholz formula. *IVS*, interventricular septum; *PW*, left ventricular posterior wall; *RV*, right ventricle.

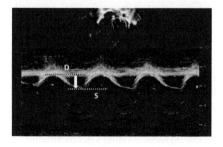

FIGURE 40

Apical four-chamber M-mode with cursor alignment through the lateral tricuspid annulus. **TAPSE** (tricuspid annular plane systolic excursion) is a parameter that corresponds to the distance (in mm) by which the lateral tricuspid annulus moves toward the apex of the heart between end-diastole (D) and end-systole (S). The higher the value, the better is the longitudinal RV systolic function. It also correlates with the global RV systolic function. Normal reference ranges are age dependant (>7−11 mm in neonates, > 15−25 mm in adults).

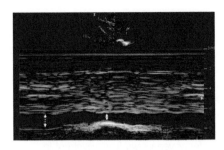

FIGURE 41

Semiquantitative assessment of the right atrial pressure based on the evaluation of the diameter and the inspiratory collapsibility of the inferior vena cava (IVC) on subcostal M-mode. Unlike in adults, age-matched IVC dimensions have not been well defined in children. More than 50% inspiratory IVC collapse (ratio between the *double arrows*) is suggestive of right atrial pressure of less than 10 mmHg.

Spectral Doppler imaging

Spectral Doppler is an imaging modality that displays blood flow velocity (in m/s) over time. In pulsed-wave (PW) Doppler, the flow velocity is recorded only from a small predefined area ("sample volume"), while in continuous-wave (CW) Doppler, the velocity curve represents all flow velocities sampled along the cursor line. By definition, a spectral waveform above the baseline represents an antegrade flow (toward the probe). The opposite is true for retrograde flow, which is below the baseline.

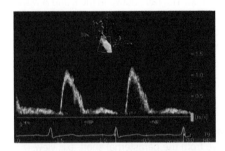

FIGURE 42

Pulsed-wave Doppler of the descending aorta from the subcostal view showing normal aortic waveform. The waveform has a "hollow" appearance reflecting the fact that the flow is laminar (all blood elements moving at a similar velocity).

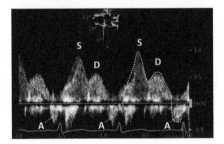

FIGURE 43

Pulsed-wave Doppler of the right lower pulmonary vein from the apical four-chamber view. The pulmonary venous waveform has three phases. The S wave represents an initial forward flow caused by the apical displacement of the mitral annulus during ventricular systole. The D wave corresponds to a second forward flow during diastolic filling of the ventricles. The S wave is normally taller than the D wave and their ratio is > 1.0. The negative A wave reflects flow reversal caused by atrial contraction.

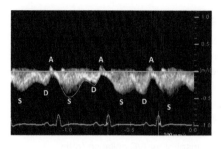

FIGURE 44

Pulsed-wave Doppler of the inferior vena cava from the subcostal short-axis (bicaval) view. Analogously to the pulmonary venous flow described above, the flow in the caval veins has also three phases (S, D, A waves). The superior vena cava flow waveform is a mirror image of the inferior vena cava flow waveform in relation to the baseline as both flows have opposite directions.

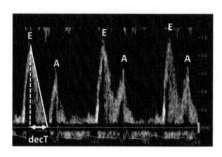

FIGURE 45

Pulsed-wave (PW) Doppler of mitral inflow from the apical four-chamber view. The waveform has two phases. The E wave corresponds to an early passive filling of the left ventricle driven by the pressure gradient between the left atrium and ventricle. The E wave ends when both pressures equalize. The A wave represents an active filling phase produced by the atrial contraction. The ratio between the E and A wave amplitudes is normally between 0.75 and 1.5, but it varies with age and heart rate. Deceleration time (decT) is the time required for the E wave to decrease from peak to zero and is between 150 and 240 ms in adults. The PW Doppler of the tricuspid inflow is analogous to the PW Doppler of the mitral inflow.

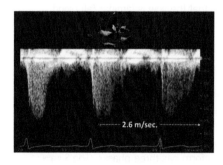

FIGURE 46

Continuous-wave Doppler of the tricuspid valve from the parasternal short-axis view. This figure shows the regurgitant signal only. The tricuspid regurgitation (TR) peak velocity allows calculation of the systolic pulmonary artery pressure using the modified Bernoulli equation. This equation is based on the fact that the gradient between the right ventricle (RV) and the right atrium (RA) is proportional to the tricuspid regurgitation (TR) peak velocity. Note that pulmonary hypertension is defined as a mean (not systolic) pulmonary artery pressure of ≥ 25 mmHg.

Systolic RV pressure—RA pressure $= 4 \times$ (TR peak velocity)^2

Systolic PA pressure $=$ systolic RV pressure $= 4 \times$ (TR peak velocity)^2 $+$ RA pressure [assumed 5 mmHg]

Systolic PA pressure $= 4 \times (2.6 \text{ m/s})^2 + 5 \text{ mmHg} = 32 \text{ mmHg}$

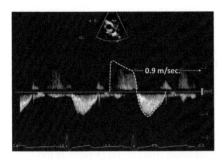

FIGURE 47

Continuous-wave Doppler of the right ventricular outflow tract from the parasternal short-axis view. The spectral waveform below the baseline represents forward flow into the pulmonary artery. The waveform above the baseline corresponds to pulmonary regurgitation (PR). Trivial PR is physiological in children. The diastolic pulmonary artery (PA) pressure can be obtained analogously to the systolic PA pressure using the modified Bernoulli equation and the end-diastolic PR regurgitation velocity.

[Assuming that right ventricular (RV) end-diastolic pressure = right atrial (RA) pressure = 5 mmHg].

Diastolic PA pressure = 4 × (end-diastolic PR velocity)^2 + RV diastolic pressure = = 4 × (0.9 m/s)^2 + 5 mmHg = 8.2 mmHg.

Systolic PA pressure = 4 × (peak TR velocity in m/s)^2 + assumed RA pressure.
Diastolic PA pressure = 4 × (end-diastolic PR velocity in m/s)^2 + assumed RA pressure.
Mean PA pressure = 1/3 systolic PA pressure + 2/3 diastolic PA pressure.

PA, pulmonary artery; *PR*, pulmonary regurgitation; *RA*, right atrium; *TR* tricuspid regurgitation.

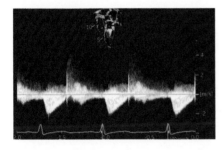

FIGURE 48

Continuous-wave Doppler of the left ventricular outflow tract (LVOT) from the apical five-chamber view. The spectral waveform below the baseline represents forward flow across the LVOT. Aortic regurgitation is an abnormal finding and is shown in this figure for illustration purposes only. The regurgitant flow waveform is above the baseline and has a high peak velocity (4 m/s) due to the systemic pressure in the aorta.

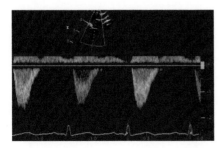

FIGURE 49

Continuous-wave Doppler of the descending thoracic aorta from the suprasternal notch view. Normal low-velocity flow waveform.

Tissue Doppler imaging

Tissue Doppler imaging (TDI) is an advanced echocardiographic technique that measures low-velocity myocardial motion. It is commonly used for assessment of the left ventricular diastolic function.

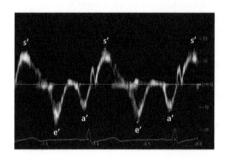

FIGURE 50

Pulsed-wave (PW) tissue Doppler at the level of the lateral mitral valve annulus showing its velocity over time. In systole, the annulus moves toward the apex of the heart, which is recorded as a positive s'-wave. In diastole, the early passive filling and the late active filling move the mitral annulus toward the left atrium. Thus, two negative waves are recorded—e' and a' waves. The peak s' wave velocity reflects the systolic function (normal value > 0.08 m/s). The E/e' ratio (E wave from mitral inflow PW Doppler/e' wave from PW tissue Doppler) can be used as a marker of diastolic function (normal value < 8). The mitral inflow PW Doppler (see Figure 44) and the measurement of the E wave amplitude are not shown in this figure.

Segmental approach to congenital heart disease

Historically, there have been two main schools of nomenclature of congenital heart defects, the foundations of which were laid in parallel by Robert Anderson from the United Kingdom and by Richard and Stella Van Praagh from the United States. For this reason, the "Andersonian" approach is used predominantly in Europe, while the "Van Praaghian" approach is more common in the United States. Despite many similarities, the two schools differ significantly in many aspects. This book is based on the Andersonian nomenclature.

The segmental approach to congenital heart disease is a multistep process in which the elementary "building blocks" that form the heart are examined. It divides the heart into three basic segments, **atria, ventricles,** and **great arteries**, and two junctions between them, **atrio-ventricular junction** and **ventriculo-arterial junction**.

The principle of segmental analysis relies on a separate identification of each cardiac segment based on the presence of key morphological criteria. These anatomical features allow the distinction between the morphological right and the morphological left atrium, the morphological right and the morphological left ventricle, and the aorta and the pulmonary artery.

It is important to understand that the spatial position of each cardiac segment plays no role in the process of their identification. For example, the term "right ventricle" refers to the "morphological right ventricle," which may, be on the right or on the left side of the malformed heart.

Another example would be the case of left atrial isomerism in which there are two morphological left atria, one on the right and the other on the left side of the heart.

The segmental approach provides an accurate way of describing congenital cardiac malformations and consists of a stepwise analysis of the cardiac position, the atrial morphology and situs, the ventricular morphology and looping, the type and mode of the atrio-ventricular connection, the ventriculo-arterial connection, and the relationship between the great arteries. Each part is discussed in a separate section below.

Atlas of Pediatric Echocardiography. https://doi.org/10.1016/B978-0-323-75981-6.00008-X

Cardiac position

The term cardiac position refers to the position of the heart and orientation of the cardiac apex in the chest (Figure 1). It is best determined from the subcostal views. In **levocardia**, the heart is situated in the left hemithorax, with the apex pointing to the left. In **dextrocardia**, the heart is in the right hemithorax and the apex is oriented to the right. In **mesocardia**, the heart is positioned in the middle of the chest, with the apex pointing to the midline. Instead of using the terms dextroversion or dextroposition, the terms dextrocardia with the apex pointing to the left or to the right, or levocardia with the apex pointing to the right should be used. The same applies to mesocardia.

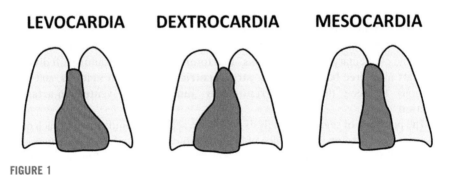

LEVOCARDIA   **DEXTROCARDIA**   **MESOCARDIA**

FIGURE 1

Cardiac positions.

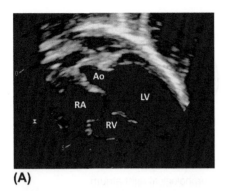

(A)

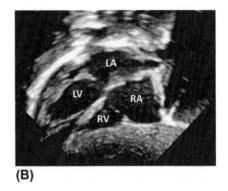

(B)

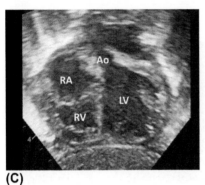

(C)

FIGURE 2

Subcostal long axis views demonstrating the cardiac position. (A) Levocardia with leftward orientation of the apex of the heart. (B) Dextrocardia with mirror image atrial and ventricular arrangement. (C) Mesocardia with midline orientation of the heart. *Ao,* aorta; *LA,* left atrium; *LV,* left ventricle; *RA,* right atrium; *RV,* right ventricle.

Atrial morphology and situs

The determination of the atrial morphology is based on the appearance of the atrial appendages. The morphological right atrium is defined by the presence of a broad-based triangular appendage, unlike that of the left atrium, which is long and narrow-based.

The term atrial situs refers to the atrial arrangement, which can be usual ("**atrial situs solitus**"—normal heart), inverted ("**atrial situs inversus**") or abnormally distributed and symmetrical ("atrial situs ambiguous"—**left atrial** or **right atrial isomerism**) (Figure 3). Apart from rare cases, the atrial situs is concordant with the thoracoabdominal situs, which describes the distribution of the asymmetrical organs in the chest and the abdomen.

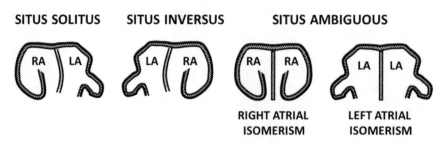

SITUS SOLITUS   SITUS INVERSUS   SITUS AMBIGUOUS

RIGHT ATRIAL ISOMERISM   LEFT ATRIAL ISOMERISM

FIGURE 3

Atrial situses. *LA*, morphological left atrium; *RA*, morphological right atrium.

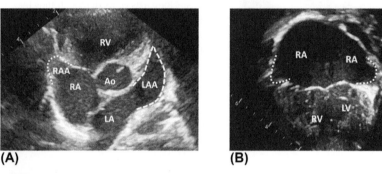

(A)

(B)

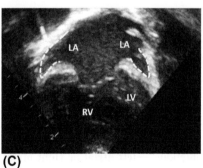

(C)

FIGURE 4

(A) Parasternal short-axis view demonstrating the shape of the right (*dotted line*) and the left (*dashed line*) atrial appendage in a normal heart. (B) Apical four-chamber view showing right atrial isomerism in a child with an unbalanced atrio-ventricular septal defect (AVSD) and other associated cardiac anomalies. Note the presence of bilateral broad-based right atrial appendages (*dotted lines*). (C) Left atrial isomerism in a patient with an unbalanced AVSD and other associated cardiac anomalies. Both atrial appendages are long and narrow based (*dashed lines*). *LA*, left atrium; *LAA*, left atrial appendage; *LV*, left ventricle; *RA*, right atrium; *RAA*, right atrial appendage; *RV*, right ventricle.

The echocardiographic identification of the atrial appendages is, however, not always practical or possible, especially in patients with poor acoustic windows. In daily practice, the determination of the atrial situs relies more on the examination of the relative position of the inferior vena cava (IVC) and the aorta in relation to the spine. The reason for this is that the suprahepatic portion of the IVC has the same embryological origin as the morphological right atrium, for which it is a good marker. The same applies to the coronary sinus. The pulmonary venous connection is, however, not a reliable marker of the morphological left atrium as it is often anomalous.

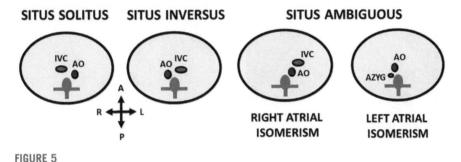

FIGURE 5

Situs identification from the position of the abdominal vessels in relation to the spine. *Ao*, aorta; *AZYG*, azygos vein; *IVC*, inferior vena cava.

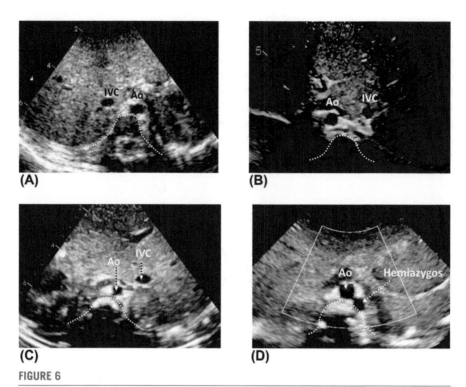

FIGURE 6

Identification of the atrial situs based on the position of the inferior vena cava (IVC) and the aorta (Ao) in relation to the spine (*dotted line*). (A) In situs solitus, the descending aorta lies to the left of the spine, the IVC is anterior and to the right of the aorta. (B) In situs inversus, the aorta is to the right of the spine and the IVC is anterior and to the left of the aorta. (C) Right atrial isomerism is characterized by both the aorta and the IVC lying on the same side of the spine. The IVC is anterior to the aorta. Both vessels are either on the right or the left side. (D) In left atrial isomerism, there is an IVC interruption with azygos or hemiazygos continuation. The aorta is anterior to the spine, the azygos or the hemiazygos vein is posterior to the aorta.

Ventricular morphology and looping

Ventricles are morphological defined by distinct anatomical features. The morphological right ventricle is characterized by coarse trabeculations, the presence of the septomarginal trabecula and chordal attachments of the atrio-ventricular (AV) valve to the interventricular septum. There is also mild displacement (offsetting) of the AV valve, which has features of the tricuspid valve, toward the apex of the heart. In contrast to this, the morphological left ventricle has a smooth endocardial surface and no chordal attachments of the AV valve, which has features of the mitral valve, to the interventricular septum.

During the early stages of embryological development, the usual rightward loop-ing of the heart tube (D—loop) leads to the morphological right ventricle being to the right of the morphological left ventricle. Leftward looping (L—loop) results in the morphological right ventricle being to the left of the morphological left ventricle. Ventricular isomerism is extremely rare because both ventricles develop in series and not in parallel.

Type and mode of atrio-ventricular connection

The step that follows the identification of the atrial and ventricular morphology is the assessment of the AV junction. The term AV connection refers to the continuity be-tween the cavity of the atrial and the ventricular chamber. In hearts with a biventric-ular AV connection, each atrium is connected to its own ventricle. Biventricular AV connections include concordant, discordant, or mixed connections. The latter case occurs in atrial isomerism.

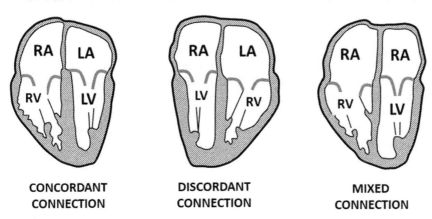

BIVENTRICULAR ATRIO-VENTRICULAR CONNECTIONS

CONCORDANT CONNECTION

DISCORDANT CONNECTION

MIXED CONNECTION

FIGURE 7

Biventricular atrio-ventricular (AV) connections (only examples with two separate AV valves are shown). *LA*, left atrium; *LV*, left ventricle; *RA*, right atrium; *RV*, right ventricle.

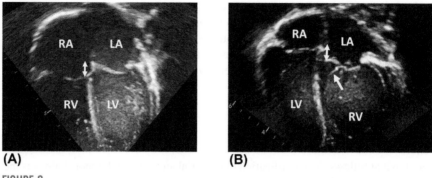

(A) **(B)**

FIGURE 8

Examples of biventricular AV connections seen from the apical four-chamber view. (A) Normal heart with concordant AV connection. The right-sided morphological right atrium connects to the right-sided morphological right ventricle. The analogy applies to the left atrium and the left ventricle. Note the presence of tricuspid valve offsetting (*double arrow*). (B) Discordant AV connection in congenitally corrected transposition of the great arteries. The morphological left ventricle is to the right of the morphological right ventricle and connects to the right-sided morphological right atrium. The *arrow* indicates the attachment of the septal tricuspid valve leaflet to the interventricular septum. The *double arrow* shows the offsetting of the tricuspid valve. *LA*, left atrium; *LV*, left ventricle; *RA*, right atrium; *RV*, right ventricle.

The term univentricular AV connection describes the connection of one or two atrial chambers to only one (dominant) ventricle. The word "univentricular" refers just to the type of connection and not to the number of ventricles. In fact, univentricular hearts commonly have a second (rudimentary) ventricle with no inlet portion. The term double inlet ventricle describes a connection of both atria to only one ventricle. The term absent right or left AV connection means that only one atrial chamber is joined to one ventricle.

UNIVENTRICULAR ATRIO-VENTRICULAR (AV) CONNECTIONS

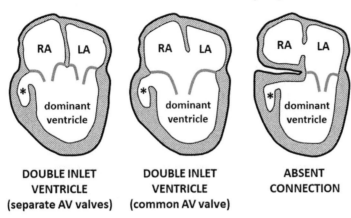

| DOUBLE INLET VENTRICLE (separate AV valves) | DOUBLE INLET VENTRICLE (common AV valve) | ABSENT CONNECTION |

FIGURE 9

Univentricular atrio-ventricular connections. Rudimentary chamber (*asterisk*). *LA*, left atrium; *RA*, right atrium.

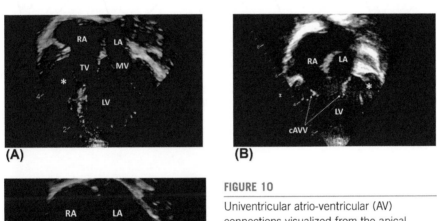

(A)   (B)

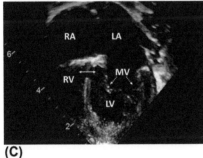

(C)

FIGURE 10

Univentricular atrio-ventricular (AV) connections visualized from the apical four-chamber view. (A) Double inlet left ventricle with two separate AV valves. Both atria connect to the dominant left ventricle. Note the presence of a rudimentary right ventricle (*asterisk*). (B) Double inlet left ventricle with a common AV valve. Both atria connect to the dominant left ventricle. The *asterisk* indicates a rudimentary (left-sided) right ventricle. (C) Tricuspid atresia with absent right AV connection. The left atrium is connected to the left ventricle, which communicates with the rudimentary right ventricle via a ventricular septal defect (*double arrow*). *cAVV*, common AV valve; *LA*, left atrium; *LV*, left ventricle; *MV*, mitral valve; *RA*, right atrium; *RV*, rudimentary right ventricle; *TV* tricuspid valve.

In addition to describing the type of AV connection (biventricular or univentricular), the morphology of the AV valves, also known as mode of AV connection, should be analyzed. Modes of connection include two perforate valves, common AV valve, one imperforate and one perforate valve and AV valve straddling and overriding.

AV valve straddling refers to an abnormal insertion of part of the valvar tension apparatus into the contralateral ventricle and is always associated with the presence of a ventricular septal defect. When there is AV valve overriding, the AV valve overrides the interventricular septum and voids into both ventricles. AV valve straddling and overriding are usually present together.

MODES OF ATRIOVENTRICULAR CONNECTIONS

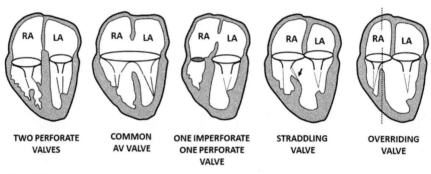

| TWO PERFORATE VALVES | COMMON AV VALVE | ONE IMPERFORATE ONE PERFORATE VALVE | STRADDLING VALVE | OVERRIDING VALVE |

FIGURE 11

Modes of atrio-ventricular connections. *LA*, left atrium; *RA*, right atrium.

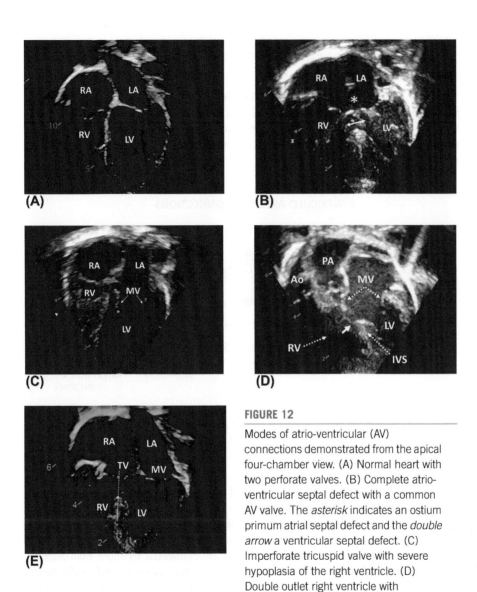

FIGURE 12

Modes of atrio-ventricular (AV) connections demonstrated from the apical four-chamber view. (A) Normal heart with two perforate valves. (B) Complete atrio-ventricular septal defect with a common AV valve. The *asterisk* indicates an ostium primum atrial septal defect and the *double arrow* a ventricular septal defect. (C) Imperforate tricuspid valve with severe hypoplasia of the right ventricle. (D) Double outlet right ventricle with ventriculo-arterial discordance. The mitral valve is overriding the interventricular septum. Note straddling of the anterior mitral valve leaflet (*arrow*). (E) Tricuspid valve overriding (*dotted line*) the interventricular septum. *Ao*, aorta; *IVS*, interventricular septum; *LA*, left atrium; *LV*, left ventricle; *MV*, mitral valve; *RA*, right atrium; *RV*, right ventricle; *TV*, tricuspid valve.

Ventriculo-arterial connection and relationship between the great arteries

This step of the segmental analysis identifies which great artery is connected to which ventricle. From the morphological point of view, the aorta is defined as a vessel that gives rise to the coronary arteries and the head and neck arteries. The pulmonary artery is characterized by bifurcation into the right and left pulmonary arteries.

VENTRICULO-ARTERIAL CONNECTIONS

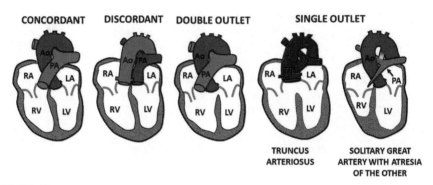

FIGURE 13

Ventriculo-arterial connections. *Ao*, aorta; *LA*, left atrium; *LV*, left ventricle; *PA*, pulmonary artery; *RA*, right atrium; *RV*, right ventricle; *TRU*, truncus arteriosus.

The following types of ventriculo-arterial connections are distinguished: **concordant** (the pulmonary artery connects to the morphological right ventricle and the aorta to the morphological left ventricle), **discordant** (the pulmonary artery connects to the morphological left ventricle and the aorta to the morphological right ventricle), **double outlet** (both great arteries are connected by more than 50% to one ventricle) and **single outlet** (only one great artery is connected to the heart, that is, truncus arteriosus, or the aorta in the case of pulmonary atresia or the pulmonary artery in the case of aortic atresia).

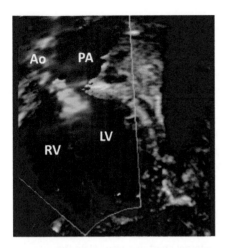

FIGURE 14

Subcostal short-axis view illustrating concordant ventriculo-arterial connection. The pulmonary artery arises from the right ventricle and the aorta from the left ventricle. *Ao*, aorta; *LV*, left ventricle; *PA*, pulmonary artery; *RV*, right ventricle.

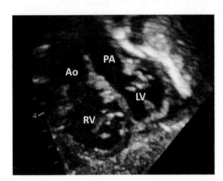

FIGURE 15

Subcostal short-axis view demonstrating discordant ventriculo-arterial connection in the transposition of the great arteries. The pulmonary artery arises from the left ventricle and the aorta from the right ventricle. *Ao*, aorta; *LV*, left ventricle; *PA*, pulmonary artery; *RV*, right ventricle.

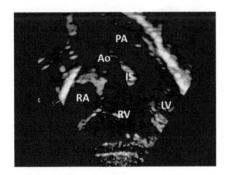

FIGURE 16

Double outlet right ventricle seen from the subcostal view. Both great arteries arise from the right ventricle. *Ao*, aorta; *IS*, infundibular septum; *LV*, left ventricle; *PA*, pulmonary artery; *RA*, right atrium; *RV*, right ventricle.

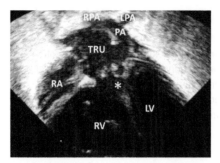

FIGURE 17

Single outlet ventriculo-arterial connection in persistent truncus arteriosus seen from the apical view. The pulmonary artery arises from the truncus. The truncal valve overrides the ventricular septal defect (*asterisk*). *LPA*, left pulmonary artery; *LV*, left ventricle; *PA*, pulmonary artery; *RA*, right atrium; *RPA*, right pulmonary artery; *RV*, right ventricle; *TRU*, truncus.

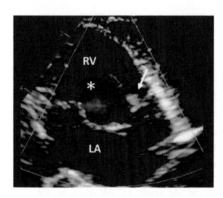

FIGURE 18

Pulmonary atresia (*arrow*) seen from the parasternal short-axis view. Note the presence of a large ventricular septal defect (*asterisk*) with an obligatory right-to-left shunt. *LA*, left atrium; *RV*, right ventricle.

The different types of spatial relationships of the great arteries are summarized in Figure 19.

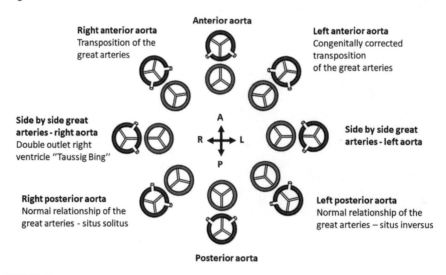

FIGURE 19

Different spatial relationships of the great arteries.

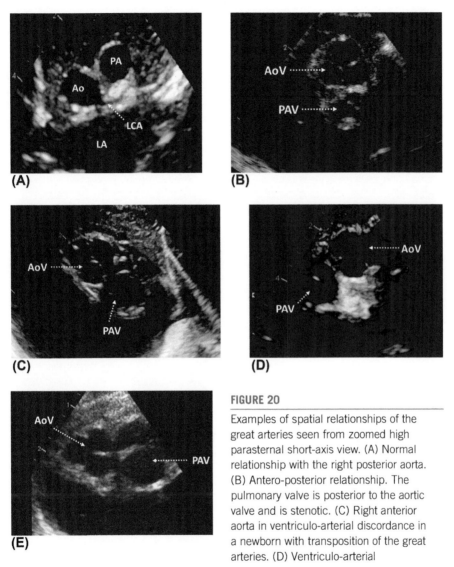

FIGURE 20

Examples of spatial relationships of the great arteries seen from zoomed high parasternal short-axis view. (A) Normal relationship with the right posterior aorta. (B) Antero-posterior relationship. The pulmonary valve is posterior to the aortic valve and is stenotic. (C) Right anterior aorta in ventriculo-arterial discordance in a newborn with transposition of the great arteries. (D) Ventriculo-arterial discordance with left anterior aorta in the congenitally corrected transposition of the great arteries. (E) Double outlet right ventricle with side-by-side great arteries. *Ao*, aorta; *AoV*, aortic valve; *LA*, left atrium; *LCA*, left coronary artery; *PA*, pulmonary artery; *PAV*, pulmonary valve.

Congenital heart defects

Atrial septal defects (ASDs)

3

The atrial septation starts with the development of septum primum, which is followed by the formation of septum secundum. Subsequently, both septae fuse and thus form the interatrial septum. This process is complex, and its disruption can lead to different types of atrial septal defects.

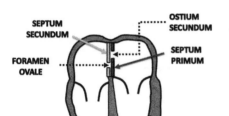

FIGURE 1

Embryological components of the interatrial septum.

Patent foramen ovale is a common finding in young children, and its overall prevalence is estimated at approximately 20% in the general population. It is a small interatrial communication, where the septum primum and secundum overlap but fail to fuse after birth, allowing shunting. **Ostium secundum atrial septal defect** is a frequently encountered anomaly characterized by an incomplete cover of the ostium secundum by the septum secundum. This is due to either excessive absorption of the septum primum or insufficient growth of the septum secundum.

Ostium primum atrial septal defect is the result of incomplete fusion between the septum primum and the atrio-ventricular endocardial cushions. This malformation falls into the spectrum of the atrio-ventricular septal defects, but is intentionally briefly mentioned in this chapter. **Sinus venosus superior** or **inferior defects** are characterized by the superior or inferior vena cava overriding the interatrial septum without its involvement. These defects are typically associated with a partial anomalous pulmonary venous connection of the right-sided pulmonary veins.

Coronary sinus defect is an abnormal communication between the coronary sinus and left atrium that is functionally equivalent to an interatrial communication. Treatment of atrial septal defects consists either in surgical, or in some patients, in transcatheter closure.

Atlas of Pediatric Echocardiography. https://doi.org/10.1016/B978-0-323-75981-6.00030-3

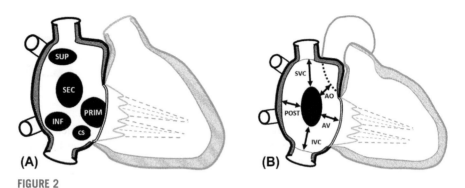

FIGURE 2

(A) Types of atrial septal defects. SEC ostium secundum atrial septal defect (ASD); PRIM ostium primum ASD (this defect does not belong to defects of the atrial septum, but to the defects of the atrio-ventricular septum and is mentioned in this figure for completeness only); SUP sinus venosus superior defect; INF sinus venosus inferior defect; CS coronary sinus defect. (B) The suitability for transcatheter closure of an ostium secundum ASD is determined by its size and the size of the rims of the septal tissue that are required to anchor the device. *AO*, rim to the aorta; *AV*, rim to the atrio-ventricular valves; *IVC*, rim to the inferior vena cava; *POST*, posterior rim; *SVC*, rim to the superior vena cava.

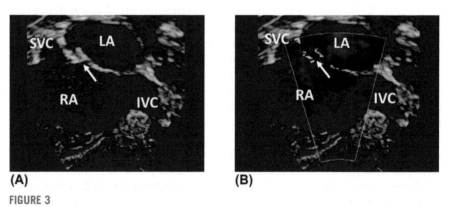

FIGURE 3

Subcostal short-axis (bicaval) view showing a small nonfusion gap (*arrow*) separating the septum primum and secundum in a patient with a patent foramen ovale (PFO). (B) Color flow mapping demonstrating restrictive shunt (*arrow*) across the PFO. *IVC*, inferior vena cava; *LA*, left atrium; *RA*, right atrium; *SVC*, superior vena cava.

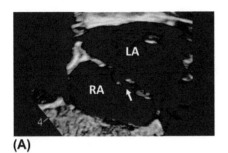
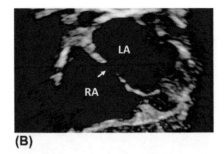

(A)   **(B)**

FIGURE 4

Difference between a patent foramen ovale and an ostium secundum ASD. (A) Subcostal four-chamber view demonstrating a patent foramen ovale. In this child, the septum secundum overlaps the ostium secundum, but there is a nonfusion gap (*arrow*) between the septum secundum and septum primum allowing a shunt. (B) Patient with an ostium secundum ASD (*arrow*). The septum secundum does not cover the ostium secundum, resulting in a defect. *LA*, left atrium; *RA*, right atrium.

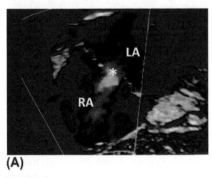
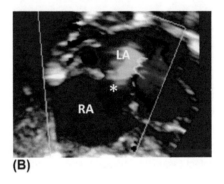

(A)   **(B)**

FIGURE 5

(A) Subcostal four-chamber view in a child with an ostium secundum atrial septal defect (*asterisk*). Note the left-to-right shunt across the defect on color flow mapping. (B) A right-to-left shunt across an ostium secundum atrial septal defect in a patient with pulmonary atresia with intact ventricular septum. The *asterisk* indicates the defect. *LA*, left atrium; *RA*, right atrium.

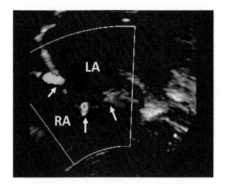

FIGURE 6

Subcostal four-chamber view demonstrating a fenestrated fossa ovalis with multiple jets of a left-to-right shunt (*arrows*). *LA*, left atrium; *RA*, right atrium.

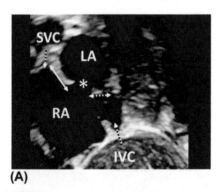

(A)

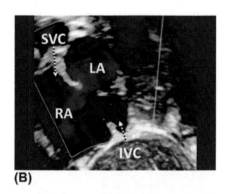

(B)

FIGURE 7

(A) Subcostal short axis (bicaval) view demonstrating an ostium secundum atrial septal defect (*asterisk*). The solid double *arrow* indicates the rim to the superior vena cava, the *dotted double arrow* the rim to the inferior vena cava. (B) Color flow mapping showing a left-to-right shunt across the defect. *IVC*, inferior vena cava; *LA*, left atrium; *RA*, right atrium; *SVC*, superior vena cava.

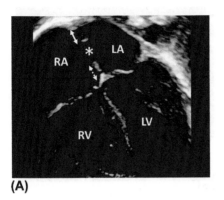

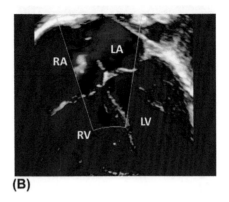

(A)   **(B)**

FIGURE 8

(A) Apical four-chamber view in a child with a moderate ostium secundum atrial septal defect (*asterisk*). *Solid double arrow* indicates the posterior rim, *dotted double arrow* the rim to the atrio-ventricular valves. (B) Note the left-to-right shunt across the defect as shown on color flow mapping. *LA*, left atrium; *LV*, left ventricle; *RA*, right atrium; *RV*, right ventricle.

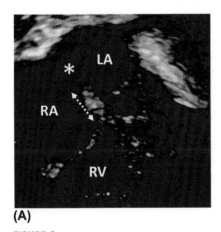

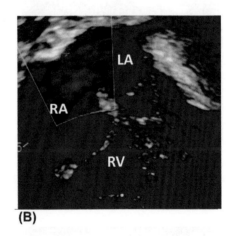

(A)   **(B)**

FIGURE 9

(A) Zoomed subcostal four-chamber view demonstrating a large posteriorly located atrial septal defect (*asterisk*) with a complete absence of the posterior rim. The rim to the atrio-ventricular valves is of good size (*dotted double arrow*). (B) Significant left-to-right shunt across the defect, as shown on color flow mapping. *LA*, left atrium; *RA*, right atrium; *RV*, right ventricle.

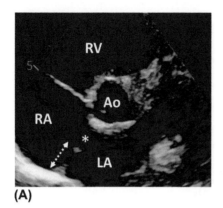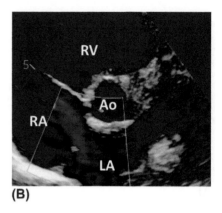

FIGURE 10

(A) Parasternal short-axis view illustrating a moderate ostium secundum atrial septal defect (*asterisk*) with absent aortic and well-developed posterior-inferior rim (*dotted double arrow*). (B) Left-to-right shunt across the defect. *Ao*, aorta; *LA*, left atrium; *RA*, right atrium; *RV*, right ventricle.

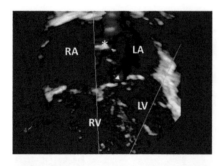

FIGURE 11

Apical four-chamber view demonstrating the difference between an ostium secundum (*asterisk*) and ostium primum (arrowhead) atrial septal defect (ASD) in a patient with an incomplete atrio-ventricular septal defect. There is a left-to-right shunt across both defects. Note that the ostium primum ASD does not belong to defects of the atrial septum, but to defects of the atrio-ventricular septum. This figure is shown for completeness only. *LA*, left atrium; *LV*, left ventricle; *RA*, right atrium; *RV*, right ventricle.

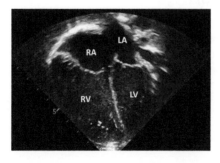

FIGURE 12

Apical four-chamber view showing severe right atrial and ventricular dilatation in a child with almost complete absence of the interatrial septum. *LA*, left atrium; *LV*, left ventricle; *RA*, right atrium; *RV*, right ventricle.

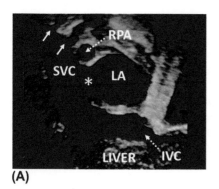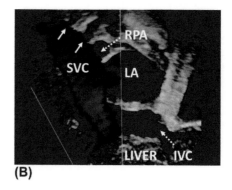

(A)   **(B)**

FIGURE 13

(A) Subcostal short-axis (bicaval) view showing a sinus venosus superior defect (*asterisk*). The superior vena cava overrides the interatrial septum. Note the anomalous drainage of the right upper and middle pulmonary veins (*arrows*) into the superior vena cava. (B) The blood flow from the superior vena cava divides between the right and left atrium, as visualized on color flow mapping. *IVC*, inferior vena cava; *LA*, left atrium; *RPA*, right pulmonary artery; *SVC*, superior vena cava.

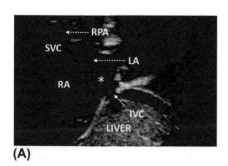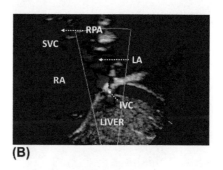

(A)   **(B)**

FIGURE 14

(A) Subcostal short-axis (bicaval) view showing the sinus venosus inferior defect (*asterisk*). Note the inferior vena cava overriding the interatrial septum. (B) Color flow mapping demonstrating flow across the inferior vena cava. *IVC*, inferior vena cava; *LA*, left atrium; *RA*, right atrium; *RPA*, right pulmonary artery; *SVC*, superior vena cava.

Courtesy of Professor Jan Marek.

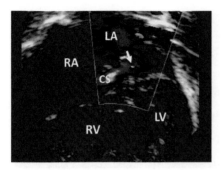

FIGURE 15

Apical four-chamber view in a child with the left superior vena cava (not shown) draining into an unroofed coronary sinus. The *arrow* indicates the abnormal shunt between the coronary sinus and the left atrium. *CS*, coronary sinus; *LA*, left atrium; *LV*, left ventricle; *RA*, right atrium; *RV*, right ventricle.

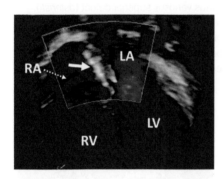

FIGURE 16

Apical four-chamber view in a child with previous transcatheter closure of a large ostium secundum atrial septal defect (ASD). The *arrow* indicates the ASD occluder device. The device has two discs that anchor it to the interatrial septum. *LA*, left atrium; *LV*, left ventricle; *RA*, right atrium; *RV*, right ventricle.

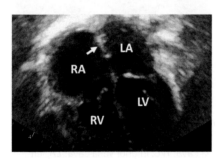

FIGURE 17

Apical four-chamber view in a child who underwent surgical closure of a large atrial septal defect. The *arrow* shows the pericardial patch closing the defect. Note the residual right atrial dilatation. *LA*, left atrium; *LV*, left ventricle; *RA*, right atrium; *RV*, right ventricle.

Ventricular septal defects (VSDs)

Ventricular septal defects (VSDs) are very common and account for approximately 20%–30% of congenital heart defects, often as part of complex lesions. From the anatomical point of view, the interventricular septum consists of a small membranous part, from which radiates a larger muscular component. The latter has three portions, an inlet, trabecular, and outlet portion.

VSDs solely affecting the membranous septum are exceedingly rare. In the vast majority of cases, membranous VSDs extend into the surrounding muscular septum and are therefore referred to as perimembranous defects. They form the largest group of VSDs. Due to a close anatomical relationship to the septal leaflet of the tricuspid valve, **perimembranous VSD**s are often restricted or even closed by accessory septal leaflet tissue. In contrast to a perimembranous outlet VSD, a muscular outlet VSD has muscular margins only. **Inlet VSD**s are typically associated with defects of the atrio-ventricular septum.

A **subarterial VSD** (or doubly committed VSD) is characterized by the complete absence of the infundibular septum and commitment of the defect to both semilunar valves. In this type of defect, the leaflets of the aortic and pulmonary valves are in fibrous continuity. In many cases, the right coronary cusp of the aortic valve prolapses into the defect, partially occluding it. This type of defect is common in the Asian population. In a **malalignment VSD**, there is a lack of alignment between the infundibular (outlet) and the trabecular septum. **Muscular VSD**s can have a variety of locations, which are summarized in Figure 1. They can occur in isolation or as multiple defects. In extreme cases, the interventricular septum has a "Swiss cheese" appearance.

Significant left-to-right shunt at the ventricular level leads to left heart volume overload, excessive pulmonary blood flow, and progressive development of pulmonary hypertension. The treatment of VSDs consists of surgical or transcatheter closure. Palliative pulmonary artery banding is performed in selected cases.

Atlas of Pediatric Echocardiography. https://doi.org/10.1016/B978-0-323-75981-6.00006-6

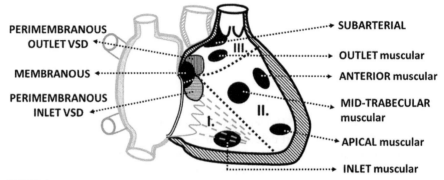

FIGURE 1

Types of ventricular septal defects (VSDs). *I.*, inlet muscular septum; *II.*, trabecular muscular septum; *III.*, outlet muscular septum.

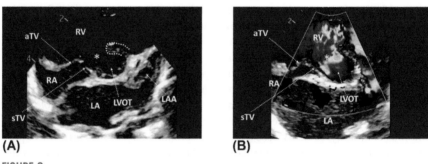

(A) **(B)**

FIGURE 2

(A) Parasternal short-axis view demonstrating a large perimembranous outlet VSD (star). The defect is near the septal leaflet of the tricuspid valve, just beneath the aortic valve. The dotted line delineates the infundibular septum. Note the dilated left atrium. (B) Unrestrictive left-to-right shunt across the defect seen on color flow mapping. *aTV*, antero-superior tricuspid valve leaflet; *LA*, left atrium; *LAA*, left atrial appendage; *LVOT*, left ventricular outflow tract; *RA*, right atrium; *RV*, right ventricle; *sTV*, septal leaflet of tricuspid valve.

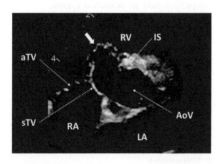

FIGURE 3

Parasternal short-axis view showing apposition of the septal leaflet of the tricuspid valve to the margins of an anatomically large perimembranous VSD, creating an aneurysmal structure. *AoV*, aortic valve; *aTV*, antero-superior tricuspid valve leaflet; *IS*, infundibular septum; *LA*, left atrium; *RA*, right atrium; *RV*, right ventricle; *sTV*, septal leaflet of tricuspid valve.

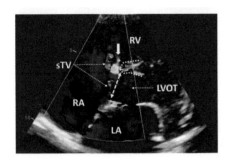

FIGURE 4

Parasternal short-axis view showing an anatomically large perimembranous VSD, which is almost completely occluded by accessory tissue of the septal leaflet of the tricuspid valve. The result is a functionally small defect. Color flow mapping illustrating restrictive shunt across the functional VSD (*arrow*). The *dashed double arrow* indicates the anatomical size of the defect. The dotted line outlines the infundibular septum. *LA*, left atrium; *LVOT*, left ventricular outflow tract; *RA*, right atrium; *RV*, right ventricle; *sTV*, septal tricuspid valve leaflet.

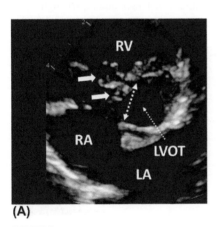
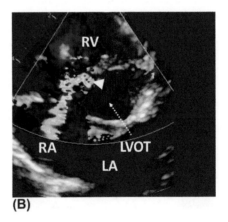

(A)   **(B)**

FIGURE 5

(A) Parasternal short-axis view in a child with an anatomically large perimembranous VSD, which is partially occluded by aneurysmal tissue of the septal tricuspid valve leaflet (*arrows*). As a result, the functional defect is much smaller. *Dotted double arrow* indicates the anatomical size of the defect. (B) Color flow mapping showing a significant left ventricular to right atrial shunt across the defect due to the incompetence of the septal leaflet. The *arrowhead* indicates the entry point of the functional defect. *LA*, left atrium; *LVOT*, left ventricular outflow tract; *RA*, right atrium; *RV*, right ventricle.

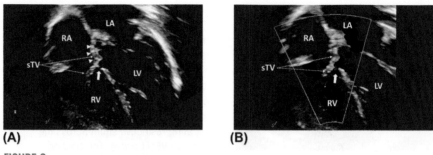

(A) **(B)**

FIGURE 6

(A) Apical view illustrating almost complete closure of a large perimembranous VSD by the septal leaflet of the tricuspid valve (*arrowheads*). As a result, the functional defect is small (*arrow*). (B) Color flow mapping showing a restrictive left-to-right shunt across the functional defect (*arrow*). *LA*, left atrium; *LV*, left ventricle.; *RA*, right atrium; *RV*, right ventricle.

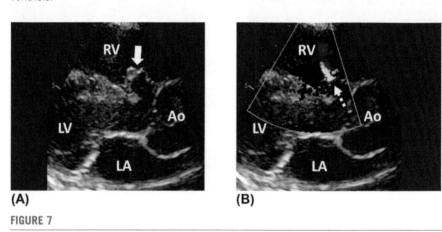

(A) **(B)**

FIGURE 7

(A) Parasternal long-axis view illustrating partial occlusion of a perimembranous VSD by aneurysmal tissue of the septal tricuspid valve leaflet (*arrow*). (B) Color flow mapping showing a restrictive left-to-right shunt (*arrow*) across the functional defect. *Ao*, aorta; *LA*, left atrium; *LV*, left ventricle; *RV*, right ventricle.

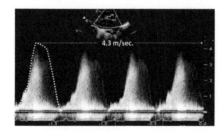

FIGURE 8

Patient from Figure 7. Continuous-wave Doppler velocity waveform demonstrating high peak blood flow velocity across the VSD (4.3 m/s), consistent with high peak systolic pressure difference between the left and right ventricle. In consequence, the diagnosis of pulmonary hypertension is unlikely in this child.

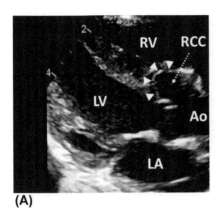 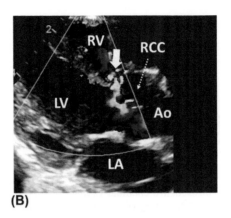

(A)   **(B)**

FIGURE 9

(A) Zoomed parasternal long-axis view in a child with an anatomically large perimembranous VSD. *Arrowheads* indicate the prolapse of the right coronary cusp of the aortic valve into the defect, partially occluding it. (B) Restrictive left-to-right shunt across the functional defect (*arrow*), as visualized on color flow mapping. *Ao*, aorta; *LA*, left atrium; *LV*, left ventricle; *RCC*, right coronary cusp; *RV*, right ventricle.

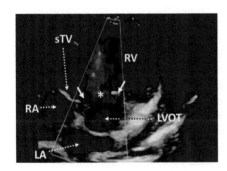

FIGURE 10

Parasternal short-axis view demonstrating a large outlet muscular VSD (*asterisk*). The *arrows* indicate the muscular margins of the defect. There is an unrestrictive left-to-right shunt across the VSD as shown on color flow mapping. *LA*, left atrium; *LVOT*, left ventricular outflow tract; *RA*, right atrium; *RV*, right ventricular outflow tract; *sTV*, septal tricuspid leaflet.

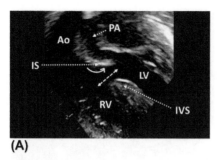 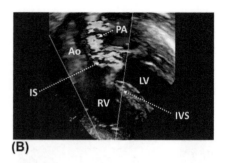

(A)   **(B)**

FIGURE 11

(A) Apical five-chamber view showing both ventricular outflow tracts in a child with a malalignment VSD (*double dashed arrow*) and transposition of the great arteries. Note the malalignment between the trabecular and the infundibular septum. The infundibular septum is deviated and protrudes into the subpulmonary left ventricular outflow tract (LVOT), causing its obstruction. (B) Color flow mapping demonstrating a systolic right-to-left shunt across the VSD and turbulent flow across the LVOT and the pulmonary artery. *Ao*, aorta; *IS*, infundibular (outlet) septum; *IVS*, trabecular septum; *LV*, left ventricle; *PA*, pulmonary artery; *RV*, right ventricle.

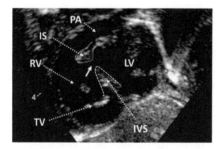

FIGURE 12

Subcostal short-axis view in a patient with tetralogy of Fallot. Note the anterior deviation of the infundibular septum (*dotted outline*), which is malaligned with the trabecular septum (*dashed outline*). The *arrow* indicates a malalignment outlet VSD. *IS*, infundibular (outlet) septum; *IVS*, trabecular septum; *LV*, left ventricle; *PA*, pulmonary artery; *RV*, right ventricle.

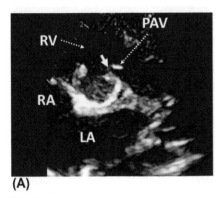 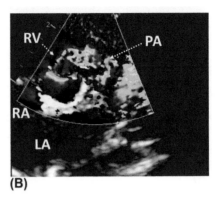

(A)   **(B)**

FIGURE 13

(A) Zoomed parasternal short axis view demonstrating a subarterial (doubly committed) VSD. The defect is located just beneath the semilunar valves. *Arrow* indicates the complete absence of the infundibular septum. (B) Color flow mapping illustrating the flow across the defect. *LA*, left atrium; *PA*, pulmonary artery; *PAV*, pulmonary valve; *RA*, right atrium; *RV*, right ventricle.

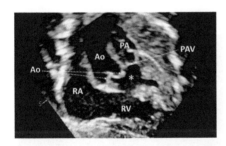

FIGURE 14

Subcostal long axis view illustrating a subarterial VSD (*asterisk*). The defect lies directly beneath the aortic and the pulmonary valves. *Ao*, aorta; *AoV*, aortic valve; *PA*, pulmonary artery; *PAV*, pulmonary valve; *RA*, right atrium; *RV*, right ventricle.

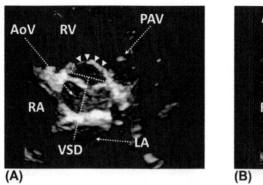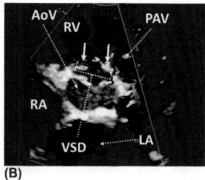

(A) **(B)**

FIGURE 15

(A) Zoomed parasternal short axis view in a patient with a large subarterial VSD. The dotted bracket shows the anatomical size of the defect. *Arrowheads* indicate a prolapse of the right coronary cusp of the aortic valve into the VSD, almost completely occluding it. Note the absence of the infundibular septum. (B) Color flow mapping demonstrating two restrictive shunts (*arrows*) around the edges of the prolapsing right coronary cusp. *AoV*, aortic valve; *LA*, left atrium; *PAV*, pulmonary valve; *RA*, right atrium; *RV*, right ventricle; *VSD*, ventricular septal defect.

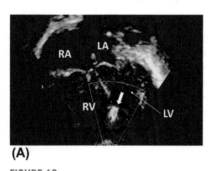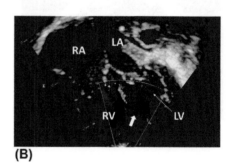

(A) **(B)**

FIGURE 16

(A) Apical four-chamber view demonstrating a midtrabecular VSD (*arrow*) with a systolic left-to-right shunt. (B) Diastolic right-to-left shunt across the defect suggests elevated right ventricular filling pressure. *LA*, left atrium; *LV*, left ventricle; *RA*, right atrium; *RV*, right ventricle.

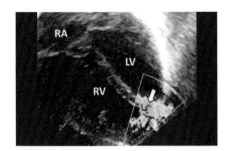

FIGURE 17

Apical muscular VSD (*arrow*) visualized from the apical four-chamber view. Note the left-to-right shunt across the defect. *LV*, left ventricle; *RA*, right atrium; *RV*, right ventricle.

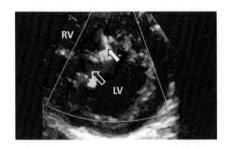

FIGURE 18

Larger anterior (*plain arrow*) and smaller midtrabecular (*hollow arrow*) VSD seen from the parasternal short-axis view. There is a left-to-right shunt across the defects. *LV*, left ventricle; *RV*, right ventricle.

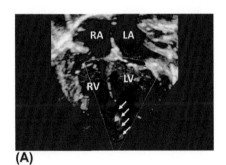

(A)

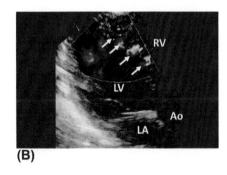

(B)

FIGURE 19

(A) Apical four-chamber view in a child with a "Swiss cheese" interventricular septum. Color flow mapping demonstrating multiple small muscular VSDs (*arrows*) with a left-to-right shunt. There is left atrial and ventricular dilatation. (B) Same heart seen from the parasternal long-axis view. *Arrows* indicate numerous muscular VSDs. *Ao*, aorta; *LA*, left atrium; *LV*, left ventricle; *RA*, right atrium; *RV*, right ventricle.

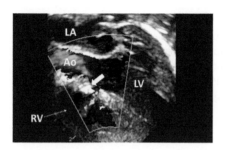

FIGURE 20

Apical long-axis view in a child with previous surgical closure of an outlet VSD. The *arrow* indicates the patch closing the defect. Color flow mapping demonstrating a small residual VSD with a left-to-right shunt. *Ao*, aorta; *LA*, left atrium; *LV*, left ventricle; *RV*, right ventricle.

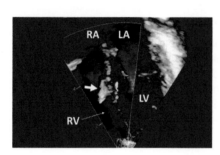

FIGURE 21

Apical four-chamber view in a patient with previous transcatheter closure of a large midtrabecular VSD. The *arrow* indicates the VSD occluder device. The device has two discs that anchor it to the interventricular septum. *LA*, left atrium; *LV*, left ventricle; *RA*, right atrium; *RV*, right ventricle.

Atrio-ventricular septal defects (AVSDs)

5

The term "defects of the atrio-ventricular septum" (AVSDs) refers to a variety of cardiac anomalies characterized by the presence of a **common atrio-ventricular (AV) junction**. This key morphological feature differentiates AVSDs from other cardiac malformations where separate left and right AV junctions are present. Depending on whether there is a fusion of the bridging leaflets of the common AV valve, the latter has either a **single common** or **two separate orifices** within the common AV junction.

Other associated features include the presence of a **trifoliate left AV valve** with a zone of apposition (the term "cleft" is inaccurate) and an **unwedged aorta.** Abnormal position of the aortic annulus, which instead of being "wedged" between the mitral and tricuspid annuli is displaced anteriorly by the common AV valve. This results in an elongation of the left ventricular outflow tract. The spatial relationship between the atrial and ventricular septae and the bridging leaflets of the common AV valve determines whether there is a shunt at atrial and/or ventricular level. In rare cases of spontaneous AV septal defect closure, there is no shunt at any level and only an isolated trifoliate valve is present.

Despite some inaccuracies and limitations, the classification of AVSDs into a complete, partial, and transitional form (Figure 1) is intentionally used in this book for simplicity. **Complete AVSD** is characterized by a single orifice of the common AV valve, the presence of an ostium primum atrial septal defect (ASD) and usually an unrestrictive inlet ventricular septal defect (VSD). In **partial** (or incomplete) **AVSD,** the common AV valve has two separate orifices due to partial fusion of the bridging leaflets. The left AV valve is trifoliate. The attachment of the fused bridging leaflets to the crest of the interventricular or interatrial septum (or rarely both) results in an isolated shunt at atrial or ventricular level (or rarely no shunt).

In **transitional** AVSD, the common AV valve has two separate orifices due to partial fusion of the bridging leaflets. The atrial component is usually large. The ventricular component is functionally restricted by aneurysmal AV valve tissue and dense chordal attachments extending from the AV valve to the crest of the interventricular septum. This form is anatomically close to a complete AVSD, but the physiology is more akin to a partial AVSD.

AVSDs account for approximately 5% of congenital heart defects and are very frequent in patients with Down syndrome. They are often associated with other anomalies such as atrial isomerism, double outlet right ventricle and tetralogy of Fallot. Corrective cardiac surgery represents the only treatment in patients with AVSDs.

Atlas of Pediatric Echocardiography. https://doi.org/10.1016/B978-0-323-75981-6.00027-3

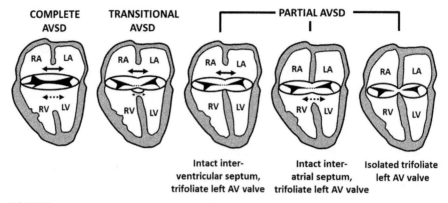

FIGURE 1

Classification of atrio-ventricular septal defects. The *double plain arrow* indicates the atrial component, the *double dotted arrow* the ventricular component. *AV*, atrio-ventricular; *LV*, left ventricle; *RA*, right atrium; *RV*, right ventricle.

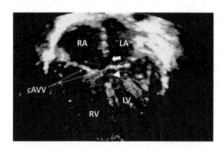

FIGURE 2

Complete AVSD with a relatively small atrial and ventricular component seen from the apical four-chamber view. The *arrow* indicates an ostium primum atrial septal defect. The arrowhead points at an inlet ventricular septal defect. The common atrio-ventricular (AV) valve has a single line appearance with no offset of the AV valves. *cAVV*, common AV valve; *LA*, left atrium; *LV*, left ventricle; *RA*, right atrium; *RV*, right ventricle.

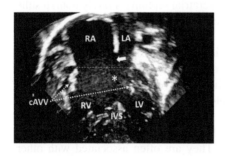

FIGURE 3

Apical four-chamber view illustrating diastolic opening of a common atrio-ventricular (AV) valve in a child with complete AVSD and a very large ventricular component (asterisk). Thin dashed line indicates the annular plane of the common AV valve. The *arrow* denotes the atrial component. *cAVV*, common AV valve; *IVS*, trabecular septum; *LA*, left atrium; *LV*, left ventricle; *RA*, right atrium; *RV*, right ventricle.

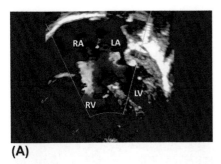
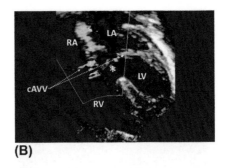

(A)   **(B)**

FIGURE 4

(A) Apical four-chamber view in a patient with complete AVSD. Color flow mapping demonstrating diastolic blood flow across a common atrio-ventricular (AV) valve. (B) Note the right and left AV valve regurgitation in systole. The asterisk indicates an inlet VSD. *LA*, left atrium; *LV*, left ventricle; *RA*, right atrium; *RV*, right ventricle.

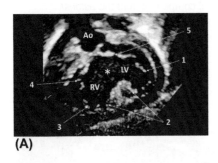
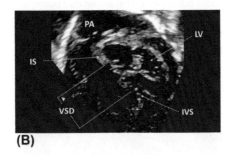

(A)   **(B)**

FIGURE 5

(A) Subcostal short-axis view in a child with complete AVSD showing the common atrio-ventricular (AV) valve en face. The leaflets of the valve are numbered (see below). Note the large ventricular septal defect (asterisk) and the origin of the aorta from the left ventricle. (B) More apical view at the level of the pulmonary artery origin from the right ventricle. En face view of the closed common AV valve in systole. Leaflets: 1 = left mural; 2 = inferior bridging; 3 = right mural, 4 = right antero-superior; 5 = superior bridging; *Ao*, aorta; *IS*, infundibular septum; *IVS*, trabecular septum; *LV*, left ventricle; *PA*, pulmonary artery; *RV*, right ventricle; *VSD*, ventricular septal defect.

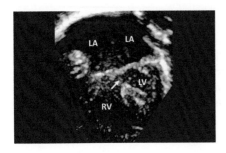

FIGURE 6

Apical four-chamber view in a child with left atrial isomerism and complete unbalanced AVSD with hypoplasia of the left ventricle. Note the small ventricular component (*arrow*) and complete absence of the interatrial septum (common atrium). *LA*, left atrium; *LV*, left ventricle; *RV*, right ventricle.

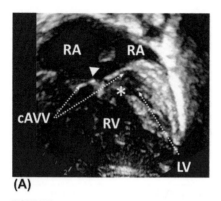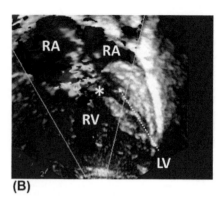

(A) **(B)**

FIGURE 7

(A) Apical four-chamber view in a patient with right atrial isomerism and complete unbalanced AVSD with a diminutive left ventricle. In addition, the child has a double outlet right ventricle with pulmonary stenosis and total anomalous pulmonary venous drainage (both not shown). The *arrowhead* points at the atrial component, and the *asterisk* indicates the ventricular component. (B) Severe right atrio-ventricular valve regurgitation, as demonstrated on color flow mapping. *cAVV*, common AV valve; *LV*, left ventricle; *RA*, right atrium; *RV*, right ventricle.

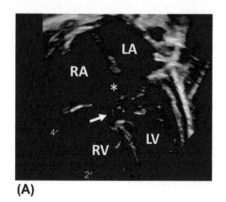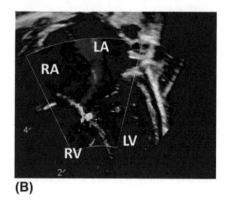

(A) **(B)**

FIGURE 8

(A) Zoomed apical four-chamber view showing a transitional form of AVSD. The aneurysmal tissue (*arrow*) of the fused anterior and superior bridging leaflets is attached to the crest of interventricular septum and significantly restricts the shunt across the ventricular component. Asterisk indicates the atrial component. (B) Color flow mapping demonstrating restrictive shunt between the two ventricles, but also left ventricular to right atrial shunt presenting as right atrio-ventricular valve regurgitation. *LA*, left atrium; *LV*, left ventricle; *RA*, right atrium; *RV*, right ventricle.

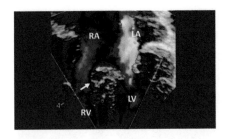

FIGURE 9

Zoomed apical four-chamber view in a patient with a transitional form of AVSD showing blood flow across the common atrio-ventricular (AV) valve. The AV valve has one annulus, but two orifices due to the fusion of the anterior and superior bridging leaflets. Note the aneurysmal AV valve tissue occluding the ventricular component (*arrow*).

LA, left atrium; *LV*, left ventricle; *RA*, right atrium; *RV*, right ventricle.

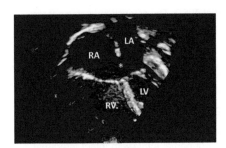

FIGURE 10

Partial AVSD seen from the apical four-chamber view. The asterisk indicates the ostium primum atrial septal defect. The interventricular septum is intact and there is no offset of the atrio-ventricular (AV) valves. The zone of apposition of the left AV valve is not shown in this figure. *LA*, left atrium; *LV*, left ventricle; *RA*, right atrium; *RV*, right ventricle.

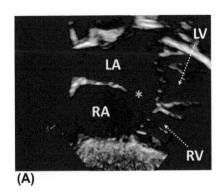
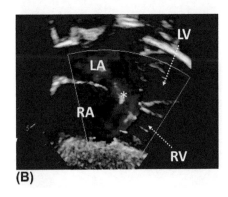

(A)   **(B)**

FIGURE 11

(A) Subcostal four-chamber view showing a detail of the interatrial septum in a child with partial AVSD. The asterisk indicates the ostium primum atrial septal defect (ASD). The common atrio-ventricular (AV) valve adhers to the crest of the interventricular septum, which is intact. Note the lack of AV valve offset. (B) Color flow mapping demonstrating a left-to-right shunt across the ostium primum ASD (asterisk). *LA*, left atrium; *LV*, left ventricle; *RA*, right atrium; *RV*, right ventricle.

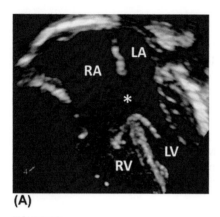 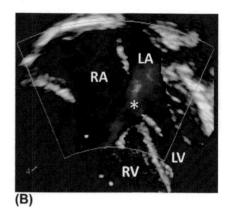

(A) **(B)**

FIGURE 12

(A) Apical four-chamber view in a child with a partial AVSD. The asterisk indicates a large ostium primum atrial septal defect. (B) Note the left-to-right shunt across the defect resulting in right atrial and ventricular dilatation. *LA*, left atrium; *LV*, left ventricle; *RA*, right atrium; *RV*, right ventricle.

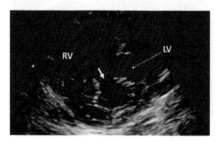

FIGURE 13

Apical four-chamber view showing a rare form of partial AVSD with intact interatrial septum and an isolated ventricular component (asterisk). *LA*, left atrium; *LV*, left ventricle; *RA*, right atrium; *RV*, right ventricle.

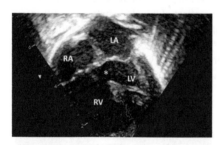

FIGURE 14

Zone of apposition (*arrow*) of the left atrio-ventricular valve seen from the parasternal short-axis view. *LV*, left ventricle; *RV*, right ventricle.

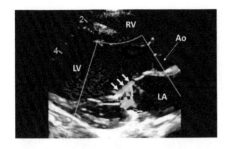

FIGURE 15

Parasternal long-axis view with color flow mapping illustrating left atrio-ventricular valve regurgitation through the open zone of apposition. Note the broad-based regurgitant jet (*arrows*). The interatrial and interventricular septae are intact in this patient. *Ao*, aorta; *LA*, left atrium; *LV*, left ventricle; *RV*, right ventricle.

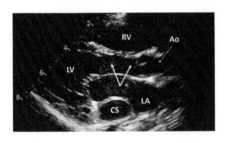

FIGURE 16

In a normal heart, the aortic annulus is "wedged" between the mitral and tricuspid annuli. In AVSD, however, the left ventricular outflow tract (LVOT) is in an "unwedged" position due to its anterior displacement caused by the common atrio-ventricular valve. As a result, the LVOT has an elongated appearance (*arrows*). This figure also shows dilatation of the coronary sinus due to the drainage of the left superior vena cava. *Ao*, aorta; *CS*, coronary sinus; *LA*, left atrium; *LV*, left ventricle; *RV*, right ventricle.

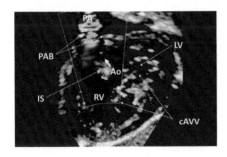

FIGURE 17

Subcostal short-axis view in a child with complete AVSD and pulmonary artery band. Pulmonary artery banding is performed in selected patients whom corrective surgery needs to be delayed. By limiting the pulmonary blood flow, the band protects the pulmonary vasculature. Color flow mapping demonstrating turbulent flow starting at the level of the band. *Ao*, aorta; *cAVV*, common AV valve; *IS*, infundibular septum; *LV*, left ventricle; *PA*, pulmonary artery; *PAB*, pulmonary artery band; *RV*, right ventricle.

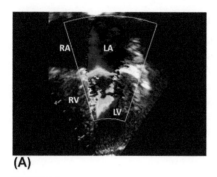

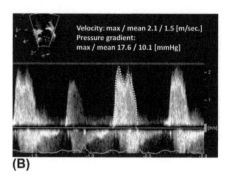

(A) **(B)**

FIGURE 18

(A) Zoomed apical four-chamber view in a child with complete AVSD and left atrio-ventricular (AV) valve dysplasia after corrective surgery. Color flow mapping illustrating turbulent flow across the left AV valve caused by residual postoperative stenosis. (B) Continuous-wave Doppler of the left AV valve inflow demonstrating an increased transvalvar pressure gradient (dotted line) of 17.6/10.1 mmHg (peak/mean gradient). *LA*, left atrium; *LV*, left ventricle; *RA*, right atrium; *RV*, right ventricle.

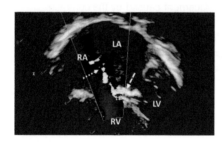

FIGURE 19

Surgically repaired partial AVSD seen from the apical four-chamber view. *Dotted arrow* indicates a pericardial patch closing the ostium primum atrial septal defect. Color flow mapping shows no residual shunt across the interatrial septum. The dashed arrow points at the sutured zone of apposition giving the left atrio-ventricular valve a thickened appearance. *LA*, left atrium; *LV*, left ventricle; *RA*, right atrium; *RV*, right ventricle.

Diseases of the mitral valve

6

The mitral valve is a complex structure that consists of several components, each of which plays a fundamental role in its function. These include the mitral annulus, anterior and posterior leaflets, chordae tendineae, and papillary muscles. The function of the valve may also be affected by anomalies of the left atrium and ventricle, for example, mitral regurgitation caused by left atrial dilatation or papillary muscle dysfunction due to ischemia of the surrounding left ventricular myocardium.

Mitral valve prolapse, isolated cleft of the anterior mitral valve leaflet, double orifice mitral valve, and **supravalvar mitral membrane** are the most common abnormalities affecting the mitral valve leaflets. **Mitral valve straddling** and **parachute mitral valve** are examples of anomalies of the tensor apparatus. Rheumatic heart disease is the most common cause of acquired mitral valve disease and is an important source of morbidity and mortality in pediatric patients in developing countries.

From a functional point of view, mitral valve abnormalities can lead to varying degrees of regurgitation or stenosis. Due to the critical importance of the mitral valve, these disorders are typically clinically poorly tolerated. Cardiac surgery is the treatment of choice in patients with mitral valve disease, but despite recent advances in valve preserving surgical techniques, mitral valve replacement may often represent the only treatment option.

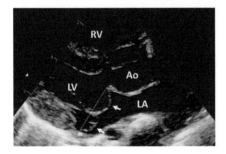

FIGURE 1

Parasternal long-axis view demonstrating severe mitral valve prolapse (*arrows*). The *dotted line* indicates the plane of the mitral annulus. *Ao,* aorta; *LA,* left atrium; *LV,* left ventricle; *RV,* right ventricle.

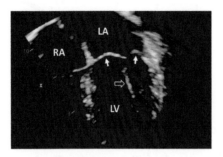

FIGURE 2

Apical four-chamber view illustrating mitral valve prolapse (*white arrows*) in a child with mild mitral stenosis. Note the thickened chordae tendineae (*hollow arrow*). *LA*, left atrium; *LV*, left ventricle; *RA*, right atrium.

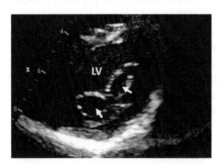

FIGURE 3

Double orifice mitral valve seen from the parasternal short-axis view. The valve is divided into two anatomically separate orifices (*arrows*). *LV*, left ventricle.

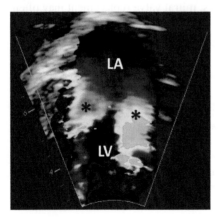

FIGURE 4

Apical two-chamber view with color flow mapping in a patient with a double orifice mitral valve. Note the division of the blood flow in two separate streams (*asterisks*), each passing through a different orifice. *LA*, left atrium; *LV*, left ventricle.

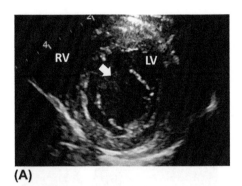

(A)

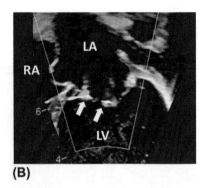

(B)

FIGURE 5

(A) Parasternal short-axis view demonstrating an isolated cleft of the anterior mitral valve leaflet (*white arrow*). (B) Zoomed apical four-chamber view with color flow mapping showing two jets of mitral regurgitation (*arrows*) across the cleft. Note the absence of an atrial or ventricular septal defect in this patient. *LA*, left atrium; *LV*, left ventricle; *RA*, right atrium; *RV*, right ventricle.

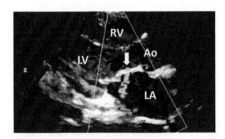

FIGURE 6

Patient after surgical repair of an isolated cleft of the anterior mitral valve leaflet. The *arrow* indicates a mild, posteriorly directed jet of residual mitral regurgitation across the anterior leaflet (at the level of the sutured cleft). *Ao*, aorta; *LA*, left atrium; *LV*, left ventricle; *RV*, right ventricle.

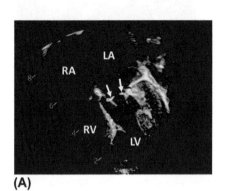

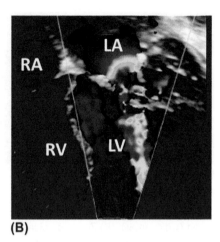

(A)   **(B)**

FIGURE 7

(A) Apical four-chamber view demonstrating a supravalvar mitral membrane (*arrows*). The membrane adheres firmly to the valve leaflets, which thus become restricted in motion. As a result, the valve orifice area is significantly reduced. Note the severe left atrial dilatation. (B) In supravalvar mitral membrane, the color Doppler aliasing starts at the level of the mitral annulus as opposed to valvar mitral stenosis, where it begins below the level of the mitral annulus. *LA*, left atrium; *LV*, left ventricle; *RA*, right atrium; *RV*, right ventricle.

(A and B) Courtesy of Professor Jan Marek.

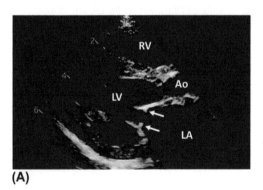

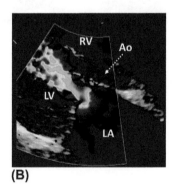

(A)   **(B)**

FIGURE 8

(A) Same patient as in Figure 7. Parasternal long-axis view showing the supravalvar mitral membrane (*arrows*). (B) Color flow mapping demonstrating turbulent flow starting at the level of the membrane. *Ao*, aorta; *LA*, left atrium; *LV*, left ventricle; *RV*, right ventricle.

(A and B) Courtesy of Professor Jan Marek.

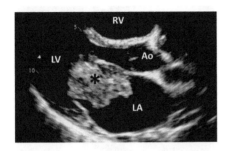

FIGURE 9

Parasternal long-axis view showing a large left atrial myxoma (asterisk) prolapsing into the left ventricle in diastole. The tumor causes significant obstruction to mitral inflow. *Ao*, aorta; *LA*, left atrium; *LV*, left ventricle; *RV*, right ventricle.

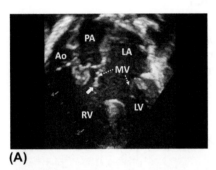

(A)

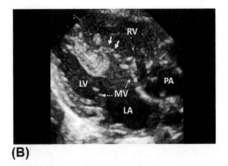

(B)

FIGURE 10

(A) Overriding and straddling mitral valve seen from the apical four-chamber view in a patient with double outlet right ventricle and ventriculo-arterial discordance. The *arrow* denotes the anterior mitral valve leaflet. (B) Same anomaly seen from the parasternal long-axis view. The valve is overriding the interventricular septum. *Arrows* indicate attachment of the anterior mitral valve leaflet to the right ventricle (straddling). *Ao*, aorta; *LA*, left atrium; *LV*, left ventricle; *PA*, pulmonary artery; *RV*, right ventricle.

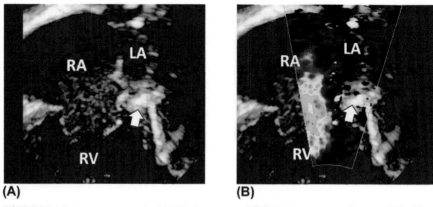

FIGURE 11

Zoomed apical four-chamber view in a neonate with hypoplastic left heart syndrome. (A) The *arrow* indicates an atretic mitral valve. (B) There is no evidence of flow across the valve (*arrow*) on color flow mapping. *LA*, left atrium; *RA*, right atrium; *RV*, right ventricle.

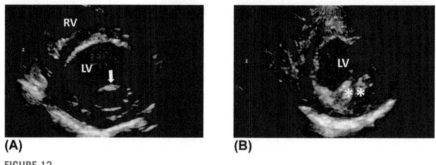

FIGURE 12

(A) Parasternal short-axis view in a child with parachute mitral valve. Note the "fish mouth" appearance of the valve (*arrow*), consistent with a small orifice area. (B) Same anomaly seen from a more apical plane. The fusion of the two papillary muscles (*asterisks*) creates a single point of attachment for the chordae tendineae. *LV*, left ventricle; *RV*, right ventricle.

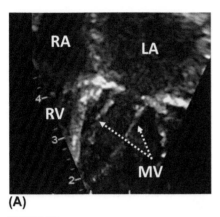
(A)

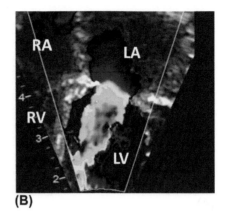
(B)

FIGURE 13

(A) Zoomed apical four-chamber view in a patient with a severely stenotic parachute mitral valve. The mitral annulus is hypoplastic and the chordae tendineae insert into a solitary papillary muscle. (B) Color flow mapping demonstrating turbulent flow across the valve. *LA*, left atrium; *LV*, left ventricle; *RA*, right atrium; *RV*, right ventricle.

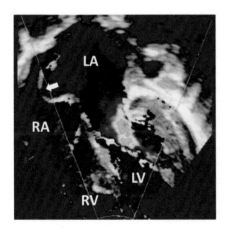

FIGURE 14

Apical four-chamber view in a child with severe mitral stenosis demonstrating turbulent flow across the valve. Due to the high left atrial pressure, there is bowing of the interatrial septum into the right atrium (*arrow*). *LA*, left atrium; *LV*, left ventricle; *RA*, right atrium; *RV*, right ventricle.

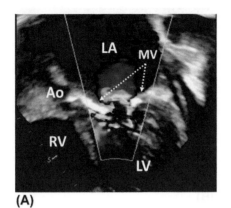 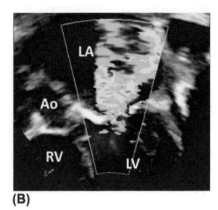

(A) **(B)**

FIGURE 15

(A) Zoomed apical five-chamber view in a patient with end-stage rheumatic heart disease and mitral valve involvement. There is severe mitral stenosis with thickening and scarring of the leaflets. The valve barely opens in diastole, which results in a significant reduction in the valve orifice area and turbulent flow. (B) Color flow mapping demonstrating severe mitral regurgitation with a broad-based regurgitant jet reaching the back of the left atrium. *Ao*, aorta; *LA*, left atrium; *LV*, left ventricle; *MV*, mitral valve; *RA*, right atrium.

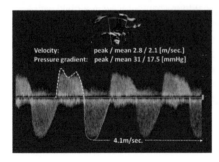

FIGURE 16

Same patient as in Figure 14. Continuous wave Doppler of the mitral valve. The transmitral pressure gradient (*dashed line*) is significantly increased (32 peak gradient, 17.5 mmHg mean gradient), indicating severe mitral stenosis. The *dotted line* represents the regurgitant signal. The peak regurgitant velocity is high (4.1 m/s) due to the systemic pressure in the left ventricle.

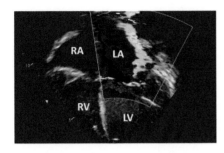

FIGURE 17

Apical four-chamber view in a patient with dilated cardiomyopathy and severe mitral regurgitation caused by incomplete coaptation of the leaflets due to dilatation of the mitral annulus. *LA*, left atrium; *LV*, left ventricle; *RA*, right atrium; *RV*, right ventricle.

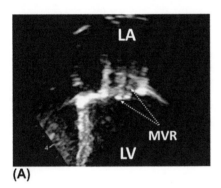

(A)

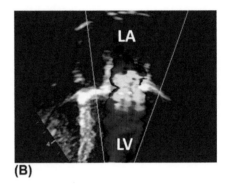

(B)

FIGURE 18

(A) Zoomed apical four-chamber view showing a prosthetic mitral valve. In diastole, the leaflets are in a parallel position allowing left ventricular filling. (B) Mitral inflow through three separate orifices in demonstrated in bileaflet prosthetic valve on color flow mapping. *LA*, left atrium; *LV*, left ventricle; *MVR*, prosthetic mitral valve.

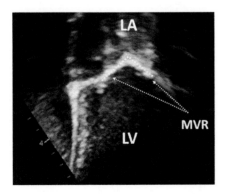

FIGURE 19

Same patient as in Figure 17 seen from a zoomed apical four-chamber view. The prosthetic mitral valve is in a closed position. The leaflets (*dotted lines*) are symmetrical and form an obtuse angle. *LA*, left atrium; *LV*, left ventricle; *MVR*, prosthetic mitral valve.

Diseases of the tricuspid valve

Diseases of the tricuspid valve form a wide range of anomalies that range from benign to critical conditions. Some of these malformations are unsuitable for the creation of a biventricular circulation. **Tricuspid atresia** is a rare defect characterized by either an absent right atrio-ventricular connection, with the right atrium and ventricle completely disconnected by the atrio-ventricular sulcus, or an imperforate tricuspid valve.

The key features of **Ebstein's anomaly** are the underdevelopment of the septal leaflet of the tricuspid valve, septal leaflet displacement toward the apex of the heart and in many patients spiral displacement of the septal and anterosuperior leaflet toward the right ventricular outflow tract. In more severe forms of the disease, the inferior leaflet is also affected and often undeveloped. The antero-superior leaflet is usually elongated, tethered to the right ventricular free wall and may have fenestrations. In some cases, the functional right ventricle is very hypoplastic due to the presence of a large atrialized portion. Significant tricuspid regurgitation and right ventricular dysfunction are often present.

Tricuspid valve dysplasia is an umbrella term for a range of abnormalities characterized by malformed tricuspid valve leaflets, chordae tendineae, and papillary muscles, resulting in tricuspid regurgitation rather than stenosis. **Overriding** and/ or **straddling** of the tricuspid valve is generally associated with complex cardiac defects. Acquired tricuspid valve disease is rarely seen in patients with rheumatic heart disease or after previous cardiac interventions.

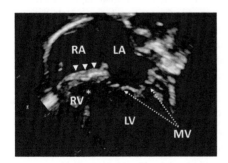

FIGURE 1

Tricuspid atresia with absent right atrio-ventricular connection (*arrowheads*) seen from the apical four-chamber view. The systemic left ventricle is connected with the rudimentary right ventricle through a ventricular septal defect (*asterisk*). *LA*, left atrium; *LV*, left ventricle; *MV*, mitral valve; *RA*, right atrium; *RV*, right ventricle.

Atlas of Pediatric Echocardiography. https://doi.org/10.1016/B978-0-323-75981-6.00010-8

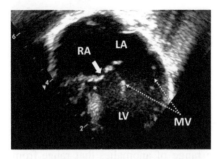

FIGURE 2

Apical four-chamber view in a child with an imperforate tricuspid valve. Unlike the mitral valve, the tricuspid valve remains closed in diastole. The *asterisk* indicates a ventricular septal defect. *LA*, left atrium; *LV*, left ventricle; *MV*, mitral valve; *RA*, right atrium.

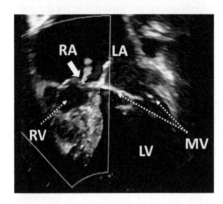

FIGURE 3

Apical four-chamber view showing a dysplastic tricuspid valve in a child with pulmonary atresia with intact ventricular septum. The right ventricle is very diminutive. There is thickening of the leaflets and hypoplasia of the tricuspid annulus. Color flow mapping illustrating trivial tricuspid regurgitation (*arrow*), confirming the patency of the valve. *LA*, left atrium; *MV*, mitral valve; *RA*, right atrium; *RV*, right ventricle.

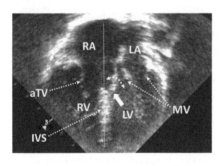

FIGURE 4

Overriding tricuspid valve seen from the apical four-chamber view. The interatrial and interventricular septae are malaligned. There is tricuspid valve straddling, with attachment of the septal leaflet to the left ventricular aspect of the interventricular septum (*arrow*). Note the large inlet ventricular septal defect (*dotted curved arrow*). *aTV*, antero-superior tricuspid valve leaflet; *IVS*, interventricular septum; *LA*, left atrium; *LV*, left ventricle; *MV*, mitral valve; *RA*, right atrium; *RV*, right ventricle.

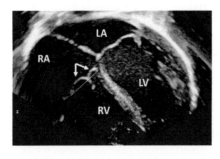

FIGURE 5

Apical four-chamber view demonstrating tricuspid valve prolapse (*arrows*). The dotted line indicates the plane of the tricuspid annulus. *LA*, left atrium; *LV*, left ventricle; *RA*, right atrium; *RV*, right ventricle.

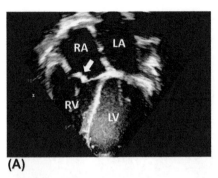
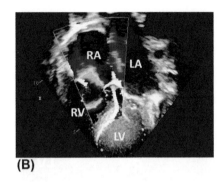

(A)   **(B)**

FIGURE 6

(A) Apical four-chamber view illustrating severe tricuspid stenosis in a patient with rheumatic heart disease. Note the thickening and scarring of the leaflets (*arrow*). (B) Turbulent flow across the significantly stenotic tricuspid valve as demonstrated on color flow mapping. *LA*, left atrium; *LV*, left ventricle; *RA*, right atrium; *RV*, right ventricle.

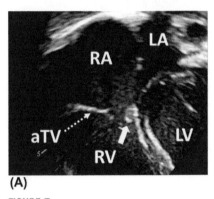
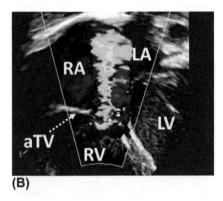

(A)   **(B)**

FIGURE 7

(A) Zoomed apical four-chamber view in a child with previous surgical closure of a ventricular septal defect (VSD). This procedure involved division and subsequent plasty of the septal leaflet of the tricuspid valve for better access to the VSD. Note the residual retraction and scarring of the septal leaflet (*arrow*), leading to an incomplete coaptation. (B) As a result, there is severe tricuspid regurgitation, as demonstrated on color flow mapping. *aTV*, antero-superior tricuspid valve leaflet. *LA*, left atrium; *LV*, left ventricle; *RA*, right atrium; *RV*, right ventricle.

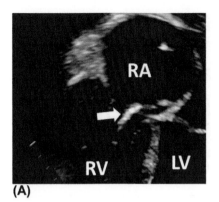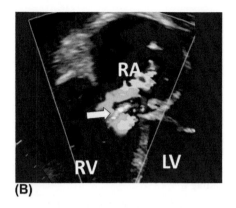

(A) **(B)**

FIGURE 8

(A) Zoomed apical four-chamber view showing an endocardial pacing lead (*arrow*) passing through the tricuspid valve in the right ventricle. (B) Severe tricuspid regurgitation caused by damage to the valve by the pacing lead. Note the right atrial dilatation. The interatrial septum is bowing to the left side, which is consistent with high right atrial pressure. *LV*, left ventricle; *RA*, right atrium; *RV*, right ventricle.

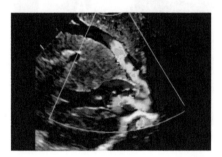

FIGURE 9

Subcostal view demonstrating systolic flow reversal in the hepatic veins in a patient with severe tricuspid regurgitation.

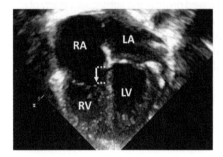

FIGURE 10

Apical four-chamber view showing a mild form of Ebstein's anomaly. The *arrow* indicates apical displacement of the septal leaflet of the tricuspid valve. The size of the atrialized portion of the right ventricle is relatively modest compared to the size of the effective right ventricle. *LA*, left atrium; *LV*, left ventricle; *RA*, right atrium; *RV*, right ventricle.

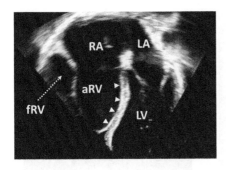

FIGURE 11

Severe form of Ebstein's anomaly seen from the apical four-chamber view. The septal leaflet of the tricuspid valve is plastered to the interventricular septum (*arrowheads*) and significantly displaced toward the apex of the heart. As a result, a large portion of the right ventricle is atrialized. *aRV*, atrialized right ventricle; *fRV*, functional right ventricle; *LA*, left atrium; *LV*, left ventricle; *RA*, right atrium.

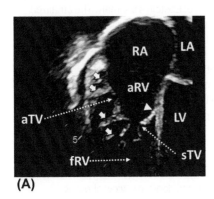

(A)

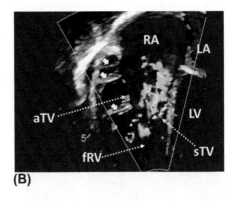

(B)

FIGURE 12

(A) Ebstein's anomaly. Zoomed apical four-chamber view showing apical displacement of the septal leaflet of the tricuspid valve (*arrowhead*). *Arrows* indicate multiple chordal attachments of the antero-superior leaflet to the right ventricular free wall. Note the lack of coaptation between the two leaflets and the thin-walled appearance of the right ventricle. (B) As a result, there is severe tricuspid regurgitation, as demonstrated on color flow mapping. *aRV*, atrialized right ventricle; *aTV*, antero-superior tricuspid leaflet; *fRV*, functional right ventricle; *LA*, left atrium; *LV*, left ventricle; *RA*, right atrium; *sTV*, septal tricuspid leaflet.

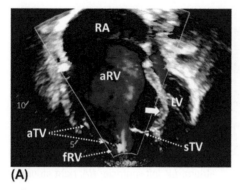
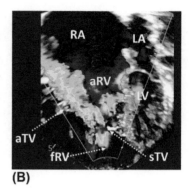

(A) **(B)**

FIGURE 13

(A) Apical four-chamber view illustrating a severe form of Ebstein's anomaly. The atrialized portion of the right ventricle is disproportionally larger than its functional portion. The *arrow* indicates diastolic bowing of the interventricular septum into the left ventricle, caused by high right atrial pressure. This reduces left ventricular filling. (B) Color flow mapping demonstrating severe tricuspid regurgitation. As a result, there is significant dilatation of the right atrium and the atrialized right ventricle. *aRV*, atrialized right ventricle; *aTV*, antero-superior tricuspid leaflet; *fRV*, functional right ventricle; *LA*, left atrium; *LV*, left ventricle; *RA*, right atrium; *sTV*, septal tricuspid leaflet.

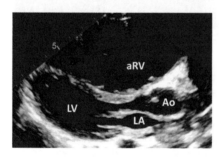

FIGURE 14

Parasternal long-axis view showing significant left ventricular compression caused by dilatation of the atrialized portion of the right ventricle in a patient with a severe form of Ebstein's anomaly. *Ao* aorta; *aRV*, atrialized right ventricle; *LA*, left atrium; *LV*, left ventricle.

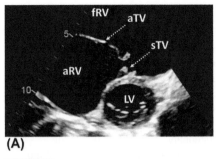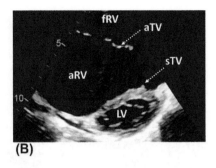

(A)   **(B)**

FIGURE 15

(A) Parasternal short-axis view (at midventricular level) in a patient with a severe form of Ebstein's anomaly. The septal leaflet of the tricuspid valve is plastered to the interventricular septum, with no effective leaflet tissue. The antero-superior leaflet is elongated and there is a large coaptation defect between the two leaflets. (B) In diastole, the interventricular septum bows into the left ventricle, compressing it. *aRV*, atrialized right ventricle; *aTV*, antero-superior tricuspid leaflet; *fRV*, functional right ventricle; *LV*, left ventricle; *sTV*, septal tricuspid leaflet.

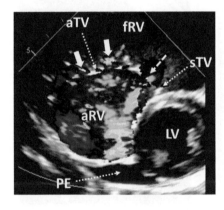

FIGURE 16

Parasternal short-axis view in a patient with Ebstein's anomaly showing an elongated antero-superior leaflet of the tricuspid valve. The leaflet has multiple fenestrations (*plain arrows*) with several jets of tricuspid regurgitation. *Dashed arrow* indicates the regurgitant jet originating from the coaptation defect between the antero-superior and the rudimentary septal leaflet. *aRV*, atrialized right ventricle; *aTV*, antero-superior tricuspid leaflet; *fRV*, functional right ventricle; *PE*, pericardial effusion; *sTV*, septal tricuspid leaflet.

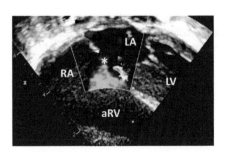

FIGURE 17

Subcostal four-chamber view illustrating an ostium secundum atrial septal defect (*asterisk*) in a child with Ebstein's anomaly. There is a right-to-left shunt across the defect due to high right atrial pressure. *LA*, left atrium; *LV*, left ventricle; *RA*, right atrium; *RV*, right ventricle.

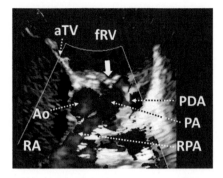

FIGURE 18

Functional pulmonary atresia in an infant with Ebstein's anomaly. Parasternal short-axis view illustrating a structurally normal pulmonary valve (*arrow*), which remains closed throughout the cardiac cycle. Color flow mapping demonstrating systolic flow in the aorta, but no forward flow across the pulmonary valve. This is due to the inability of the right ventricle to generate enough pressure to open the valve. The pulmonary blood supply is thus duct dependant. *aTV*, antero-superior tricuspid leaflet; *fRV*, functional right ventricle; *PA*, pulmonary artery; *PDA*, patent ductus arteriosus; *RA*, right atrium; *RPA*, right pulmonary artery.

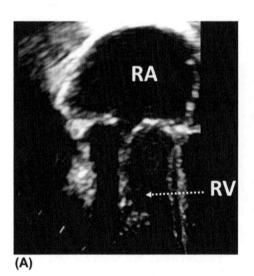
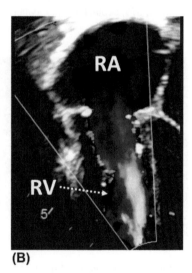

(A) **(B)**

FIGURE 19

(A) Zoomed apical four-chamber view in a patient with Ebstein's anomaly after surgical reconstruction of the tricuspid valve (cone procedure). This intervention aims to restore the anatomical position of the valve and the coaptation between the leaflets. (B) Color flow mapping demonstrating laminar blood flow across the reconstructed valve. *RA*, right atrium; *RV*, right ventricle.

Diseases of the left ventricular outflow tract

The left ventricular outflow tract (LVOT) consists of three parts, i.e., the subvalvar, valvar, and supravalvar component. Obstruction to the blood flow can occur at any level but is most commonly caused by aortic valve involvement. In the long term, turbulent flow across the LVOT can lead to aortic valve damage. In addition, an increase in afterload can result in the progressive development of left ventricular hypertrophy, dilatation, and possibly failure, accounting for significant morbidity and mortality in this group of patients. Cardiac surgery and transcatheter procedures represent the mainstay of therapy for these anomalies.

Subvalvar aortic stenosis

Obstruction of the left ventricular outflow is most often caused by the presence of a fibromuscular shelf, fibrous membrane, posterior deviation of the infundibular septum, or in patients with hypertrophic cardiomyopathy, by the systolic anterior motion of the anterior mitral valve leaflet. Less frequent causes include cardiac tumors or abnormal accessory attachment of the mitral valve to the outlet septum.

The subvalvar area is best visualized from the parasternal long-axis view, from where the etiology of the obstruction can be determined. Surgical or interventional treatment is often very demanding, and in some cases, especially in the subaortic membrane, the lesions tend to recur despite successful initial therapy.

Atlas of Pediatric Echocardiography. https://doi.org/10.1016/B978-0-323-75981-6.00021-2

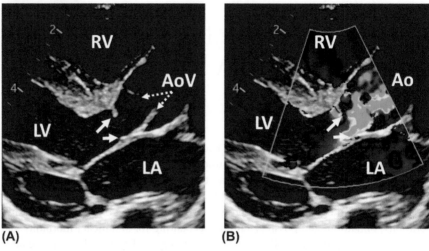

FIGURE 1

(A) Parasternal long-axis view showing a discrete circular subaortic membrane (*arrows*) and its close relationship to the anterior mitral valve leaflet and the outlet septum. (B) Color flow mapping demonstrating turbulent flow across the left ventricular outflow tract, starting at the level of the membrane. The flow turbulence is likely to cause long-term aortic valve damage, resulting in aortic regurgitation. *AoV*, aortic valve; *LA*, left atrium; *LV*, left ventricle.

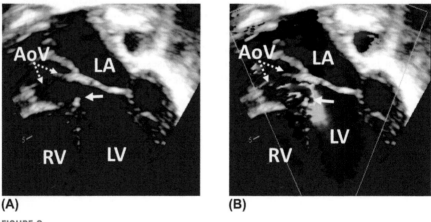

FIGURE 2

(A) Apical five-chamber view in a child with subvalvar aortic stenosis. There is a fibromuscular ridge (*arrow*) arising from the outlet septum, protruding into the left ventricular outflow tract (LVOT). (B) Color flow mapping showing turbulent flow in the LVOT caused by the presence of the ridge. *AoV*, aortic valve; *LA*, left atrium; *LV*, left ventricle; *RV*, right ventricle.

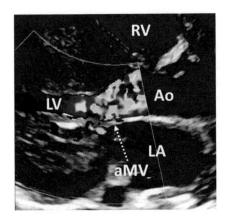

FIGURE 3

Parasternal long-axis view in a patient with hypertrophic cardiomyopathy and subvalvar aortic stenosis due to systolic anterior motion of the anterior mitral valve leaflet. The distal portion of the anterior mitral valve leaflet is displaced against the hypertrophied interventricular septum due to the Venturi effect. This results in significant left ventricular outflow tract obstruction as demonstrated on color flow mapping. *Ao*, aorta; *aMV*, anterior mitral valve leaflet; *LA*, left atrium; *LV*, left ventricle; *RV*, right ventricle.

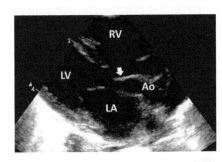

FIGURE 4

Parasternal long-axis view in an infant with interrupted aortic arch and malalignment ventricular septal defect. There is a posterior deviation of the infundibular septum (*arrow*) resulting in subvalvar aortic stenosis and reduced aortic flow. *Ao*, aorta; *LA*, left atrium; *LV*, left ventricle; *RV*, right ventricle.

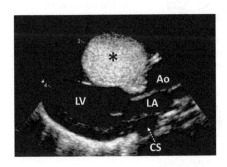

FIGURE 5

Parasternal long-axis view demonstrating a giant rhabdomyoma arising from the interventricular septum. The lesion is partially protruding into the left ventricular outflow tract, causing its severe obstruction. In this case, there was minimal antegrade flow across the aortic valve, resulting in the aortic arch being filled retrogradely from the duct. *Ao*, aorta; *CS*, coronary sinus; *LA*, left atrium; *LV*, left ventricle.

Aortic valve disease

Aortic valve disease causes either regurgitation or stenosis, and in some cases both. In children, aortic stenosis leads to a wide range of manifestations. At the extreme end of the spectrum, it is associated with major underdevelopment of the left-sided cardiac structures as seen, for example, in hypoplastic left heart syndrome. In these patients, reduced antegrade flow across the aortic valve will result in the retrograde filling of the ascending aorta and the aortic arch from the duct and dependence of the circulation on ductal flow. Associated cardiac dysfunction is almost invariably present.

Characteristic echocardiographic features of valvar aortic stenosis include thickening of the cusps, restricted cusp motion, and commissural fusion, creating a "doming" appearance of the valve in systole. The number of cusps may be variable, ranging from unicommissural to quadricommissural valves. In older children, valvar aortic stenosis is most commonly observed in association with bicommissural (bicuspid) aortic valves. Severe aortic stenosis is defined by a mean transvalvar gradient >40 mmHg. However, the gradient is irrelevant in patients with duct dependent circulation, left ventricular dysfunction, or associated lesions such as coarctation of the aorta or ventricular septal defect with a left-to-right shunt.

Aortic regurgitation is usually acquired, in particular due to previous cardiac procedures, less often congenital. Therapy for aortic valve disease includes surgical or transcatheter treatment.

MORPHOLOGY OF THE AORTIC VALVE

UNICOMMISSURAL VALVE WITH TWO RAPHES

UNICOMMISSURAL VALVE WITH TWO FUSED COMMISSURES

BICOMMISSURAL VALVE ("PURELY BICUSPID VALVE")

BICOMMISSURAL VALVE WITH ONE RAPHE

TRICOMMISSURAL VALVE (NORMAL)

TRICOMMISSURAL VALVE WITH ONE FUSED COMMISSURE

FIGURE 6

Examples of common morphological types of the aortic valve and the nomenclature. The term "commissure" refers to the point of contact between two adjacent valvar leaflets as they insert into the annulus. Uni-, bi-, and tricommissural valves are the most common. "Raphe" is a remnant of a commissure between two underdeveloped adjacent leaflets. In contrast, the term "fused commissure" is used when fusion between two initially well-developed leaflets occurs. The fusion can be either complete or incomplete. *LCC*, left coronary cusp; *NCC*, noncoronary cusp; *RCC*, right coronary cusp.

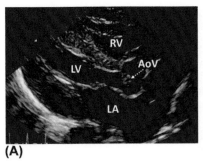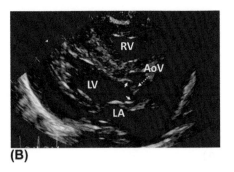

(A)   **(B)**

FIGURE 7

(A) Parasternal long-axis view in a child with severe aortic stenosis demonstrating significant thickening of the valve. (B) Due to the restricted cusp motion and commissural fusion, the systolic opening of the valve creates a "doming" appearance (*arrows*). Note the significant left ventricular hypertrophy. *AoV*, aortic valve; *LA*, left atrium; *LV*, left ventricle; *RV*, right ventricle.

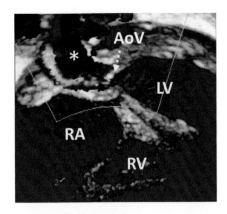

FIGURE 8

Subcostal long-axis view in an infant with critical aortic stenosis. The aortic valve is thickened and barely opens in systole. Color flow mapping demonstrates an eccentric, antegrade flow across the aortic valve. This flow is negligible compared to the ductal flow (*asterisk*) filling the aortic arch and the ascending aorta retrogradely. Note the significant left ventricular hypertrophy. *AoV*, aortic valve; *LV*, left ventricle; *RA*, right atrium; *RV*, right ventricle.

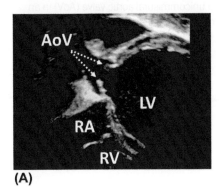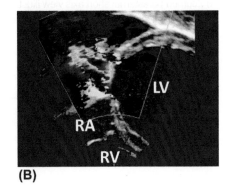

(A)   **(B)**

FIGURE 9

(A) Zoomed subcostal long-axis view in a neonate with critical aortic stenosis. The aortic valve is thickened and doming. The left ventricle is dilated, thin-walled, and severely dysfunctional. (B) Color flow mapping demonstrating turbulent flow starting at the level of the valve. *AoV*, aortic valve; *LV*, left ventricle; *RA*, right atrium.

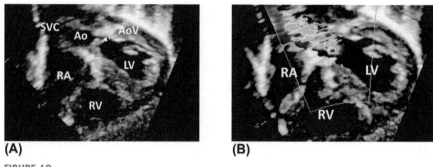

FIGURE 10

(A) Subcostal long-axis view in an infant with critical aortic stenosis. The aortic valve is severely dysplastic and thickened. There is associated left ventricular hypertrophy. (B) Color flow mapping demonstrating turbulent flow across the valve. *Ao*, aorta; *AoV*, aortic valve; *LV*, left ventricle; *RA*, right atrium; *RV*, right ventricle; *SVC*, superior vena cava.

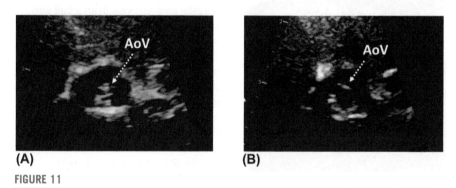

FIGURE 11

(A) Zoomed parasternal short axis view illustrating a unicommisural aortic valve (AoV) in an infant with critical aortic stenosis. (B) Systolic frame demonstrating opening of the valve.

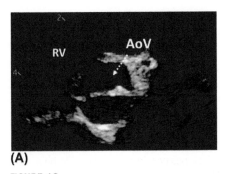 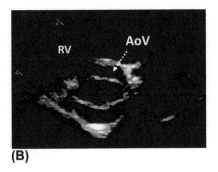

(A)   **(B)**

FIGURE 12

(A) Zoomed parasternal short axis view showing a bicommissural ("purely" bicuspid) aortic valve with two symmetrical leaflets. Note the absence of raphe. (B) Opening of the valve in systole. *AoV*, aortic valve; *RV*, right ventricle.

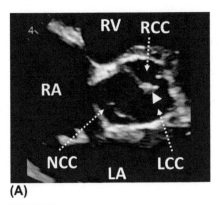 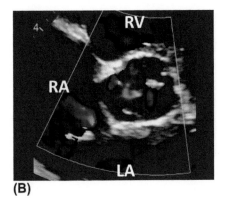

(A)   **(B)**

FIGURE 13

(A) Zoomed parasternal short axis view illustrating a bicommissural aortic valve with raphe (*arrowhead*). There is only remnant of commissure within the right and left aortic sinus. (B) Color flow mapping demonstrating blood flow across the effective orifice of the valve. *LA*, left atrium; *LCC*, left coronary cusp; *NCC*, noncoronary cusp; *RA*, right atrium; *RCC*, right coronary cusp; *RV*, right ventricle.

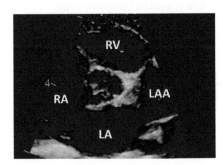

FIGURE 14

Zoomed parasternal short axis view illustrating a dysplastic tricommissural aortic valve in a patient with severe aortic stenosis. Note the significant thickening of the cusps. *LA*, left atrium; *LAA*, left atrial appendage; *RA*, right atrium; *RV*, right ventricle.

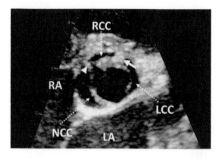

FIGURE 15

Zoomed parasternal short axis view in a child with aortic stenosis. The aortic valve is unicommisural and has one fused commissure and one raphe. The *arrowhead* at the 10 o'clock position indicates a partial fusion between the noncoronary and right coronary cusp. The thickened and dysplastic tissue at the 2 o'clock position (*arrow*) appears to be a fibrotic raphe. Both contribute to the reduction of the effective orifice area of the valve. *LA*, left atrium; *LCC* left coronary cusp; *NCC*, noncoronary cusp; *RA*, right atrium; *RCC*, right coronary cusp.

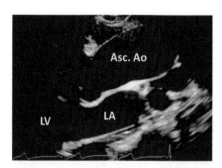

FIGURE 16

Zoomed parasternal long-axis view illustrating poststenotic dilatation of the ascending aorta in a patient with aortic stenosis. *asc.*, Ao ascending aorta; *LA*, left atrium; *LV*, left ventricle.

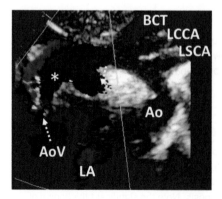

FIGURE 17

Suprasternal notch view in a neonate with critical aortic stenosis and severe left ventricular dysfunction. Color flow mapping demonstrates an eccentric, antegrade flow across the aortic valve. This flow is modest compared to the ductal flow (*asterisk*), which fills the aortic arch and the ascending aorta retrogradely. *Ao*, aorta; *AoV*, aortic valve; *BCT*, brachiocephalic trunk; *LA*, left atrium; *LCCA*, left common carotid artery; *LSCA*, left subclavian artery.

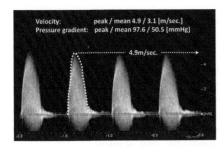

FIGURE 18

Evaluation of aortic stenosis by continuous-wave Doppler is best performed from the suprasternal notch view. In this patient with severe aortic stenosis, there is a significant increase in the peak systolic velocity of blood flow across the aortic valve (4.9 m/s), consistent with a peak and mean pressure gradient of 97.6 and 50.5 mmHg, respectively.

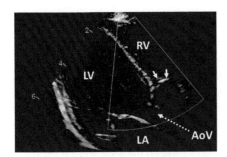

FIGURE 19

Parasternal long-axis view in a child with a large perimembranous ventricular septal defect and prolapse of the right coronary cusp into the defect (*arrows*). As a result, there is trivial aortic regurgitation, which is likely to progress in the long term. *AoV*, aortic valve; *LA*, left atrium; *LV*, left ventricle; *RV*, right ventricle.

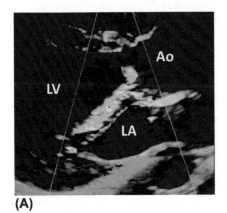

(A)

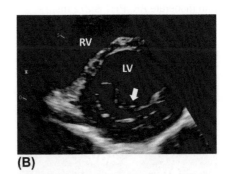

(B)

FIGURE 20

(A) Parasternal long-axis view in a patient with mild aortic stenosis and severe aortic regurgitation. Note the eccentric, posteriorly directed regurgitation jet, which displaces the anterior mitral valve leaflet toward the left atrium. (B) Parasternal short-axis view in the same patient demonstrating "banana" shaped mitral valve orifice with posterior displacement (*arrow*) of the anterior leaflet by the regurgitation jet. *Ao*, aorta; *LA*, left atrium; *LV*, left ventricle.

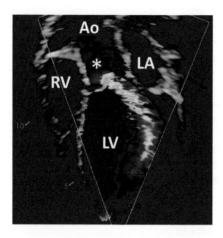

FIGURE 21

Severe aortic regurgitation seen from the apical five-chamber view. Note the broad-based regurgitation jet causing swirling flow in the left ventricle. There is a flow reversal in the ascending aorta (*asterisk*) and significant dilatation of the left ventricle. *Ao*, aorta; *LA*, left atrium; *LV*, left ventricle; *RV*, right ventricle.

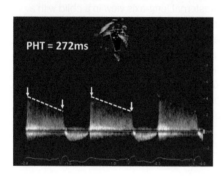

FIGURE 22

The pressure half time (PHT) of the aortic regurgitation flow velocity is a useful tool for evaluating the severity of aortic regurgitation (AR). PHT corresponds to the time needed for the maximal pressure gradient between the aorta and the left ventricle to reduce by 50% (square root relationship for flow velocity). PHT reflects the severity of AR, but also depends on the compliance of the left ventricle. PHT >500 ms reflects mild AR, while PHT <200 ms is consistent with severe AR. In this child with moderate AR, PHT is 272 ms.

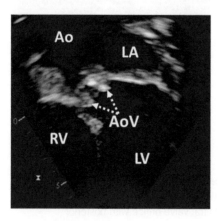

FIGURE 23

Apical five-chamber view demonstrating a prosthetic aortic valve. *Arrows* indicate leaflets of the valve. *Ao*, aorta; *AoV*, aortic valve; *LA*, left atrium; *LV*, left ventricle; *RV*, right ventricle.

Supravalvar aortic stenosis

Supravalvar aortic stenosis is typically caused by a localized narrowing of the aorta at the level of the sinotubular junction. However, instead of having a discrete stenotic lesion, a minority of children have long segment hypoplasia of the ascending aorta and the aortic arch. This anomaly occurs almost exclusively in patients with Williams syndrome, in whom the disease is observed in more than 50% of cases. Surgical repair is the only treatment.

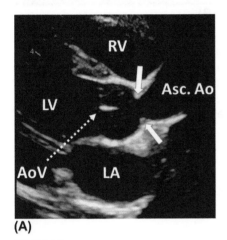 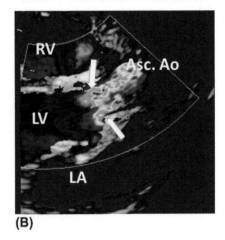

(A)   **(B)**

FIGURE 24

(A) Parasternal long-axis views in a child with Williams syndrome and supravalvar aortic stenosis. *Arrows* indicate a discrete narrowing at the level of the sinotubular junction, which produces an hourglass appearance. The aortic valve is normal. (B) Color flow mapping demonstrating turbulent flow across the sinotubular junction (*arrows*). *AoV*, aortic valve; *asc.*, Ao ascending aorta; *LA*, left atrium; *LV*, left ventricle; *RV* right ventricle.

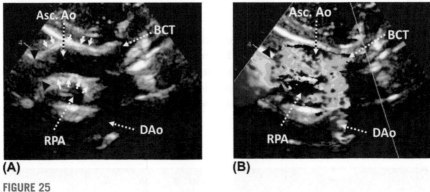

FIGURE 25

(A) Suprasternal notch view in a patient with Williams syndrome. *Black arrowheads* indicate the narrowed sinotubular junction. Note the long segment hypoplasia of the ascending aorta with thickening of the aortic wall (*white arrows*). (B) Turbulent flow across the hypoplastic ascending aorta starting at the level of the sinotubular junction (*black arrowheads*). *Asc*, Ao ascending aorta; *BCT*, brachiocephalic trunk; *Dao*, descending aorta; *RPA*, right pulmonary artery.

Diseases of the right ventricular outflow tract (RVOT)

9

Abnormalities of the right ventricular outflow tract (RVOT) belong to the most common heart defects and are often part of complex cardiac malformations. Obstruction of RVOT can occur at three different levels, that is, at subvalvar, valvar, and supravalvar level. Multilevel stenosis is not uncommon, particularly in complex defects, such as tetralogy of Fallot. Severely obstructive lesions are usually associated with a diminutive right ventricle.

The clinical picture varies considerably between different groups of patients. Critical pulmonary stenosis in a neonate typically causes a severe reduction in blood flow across the pulmonary valve, profound cyanosis, and circulatory dependence on ductal flow. At the other end of the spectrum, patients with a mild degree of obstruction are usually asymptomatic. Therapy of RVOT diseases consists in surgical or transcatheter treatment.

Subvalvar pulmonary stenosis (including double-chambered right ventricle)

Subvalvar pulmonary stenosis is most commonly present in patients with tetralogy of Fallot, whom it is caused by hypertrophy of the subpulmonary infundibulum, together with an anterior deviation of the infundibular septum. Due to its dynamic nature, the maximum of the obstruction occurs toward the end of systole when the infundibulum is most contracted. In contrast to the left ventricular outflow tract, fibromuscular membranes are not a common cause of subvalvar pulmonary stenosis.

Double-chambered right ventricle is a rare condition characterized by midcavitary obstruction caused by the presence of abnormal muscle bundles in the right ventricle. This anomaly is mentioned in this chapter for completeness only.

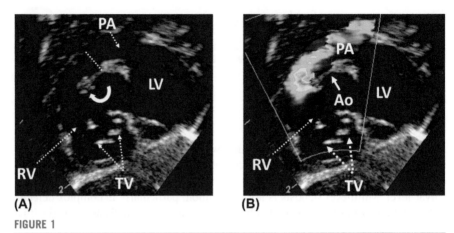

(A)   **(B)**

FIGURE 1

(A) Subcostal short-axis view in a patient with tetralogy of Fallot and mild subvalvar pulmonary stenosis. *Curved arrow* indicates the anterior deviation of the infundibular septum, which is protruding into the right ventricular outflow tract. *Dotted line* represents the level of the pulmonary valve. Note the aortic overriding. (B) Color aliasing starting at the level of the deviated infundibular septum. *Ao*, aorta; *LV*, left ventricle; *PA*, pulmonary artery; *TV*, tricuspid valve.

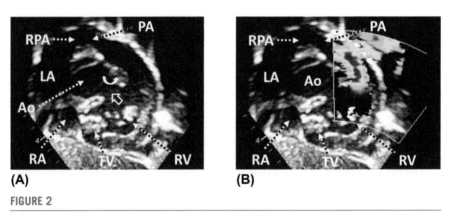

(A)   **(B)**

FIGURE 2

(A) Subcostal short-axis view in a child with tetralogy of Fallot. The infundibular septum is hypertrophied and deviated anteriorly (*curved arrow*) against the (infundibular) right ventricular free wall, causing right ventricular outflow tract (RVOT) obstruction at subvalvar level. *Hollow arrow* denotes a large perimembranous ventricular septal defect. (B) Color flow mapping demonstrating turbulent flow across the infundibulum, caused by the deviated infundibular septum. *Ao*, aorta; *IS*, infundibular septum; *LA*, left atrium; *PA*, pulmonary artery; *RA*, right atrium; *RPA*, right pulmonary artery; *RV*, right ventricle.

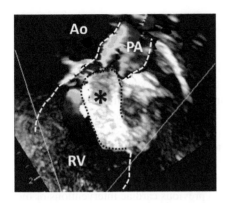

FIGURE 3

Apical view (anterior plane) in a child with tuberous sclerosis and a giant rhabdomyoma (*asterisk*) arising from the interventricular septum. The tumor causes obstruction to flow across the outlet portion of the right ventricle. *Ao*, aorta; *PA*, pulmonary artery; *RV*, right ventricle.

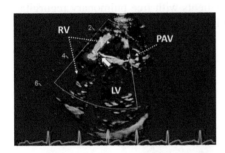

FIGURE 4

Double-chambered right ventricle seen from the subcostal short-axis view. Note the presence of anomalous muscle bundles (*arrow*) dividing the right ventricle into two parts. This results in midcavitary obstruction as demonstrated on color flow mapping. *LV*, left ventricle; *PAV*, pulmonary valve; *RV*, right ventricle.

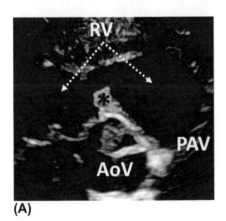

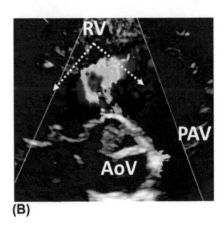

(A)   **(B)**

FIGURE 5

(A) Zoomed parasternal short-axis view in a child with a double-chambered right ventricle. The *asterisk* indicates abnormal muscle bundles partially dividing the right ventricle into two separate chambers. (B) Color flow mapping showing obstruction to flow starting at midcavitary level. *AoV*, aortic valve; *PAV*, pulmonary valve.

Pulmonary valve disease and supravalvar pulmonary stenosis

Pulmonary valve disease is either congenital or acquired. Pulmonary valve stenosis is the most common type of anomaly affecting the right ventricular outflow tract. The characteristic echocardiographic features include thickening of the leaflets, commissural fusion, systolic doming, and reduced valve orifice area. Supravalvar pulmonary stenosis rarely occurs in isolation and is generally associated with valvar pulmonary stenosis. Dominant supravalvar stenosis is typically seen in children with Noonan's syndrome (see Chapter 29).

Trivial pulmonary regurgitation can be considered physiological. In more severe cases, the regurgitation is usually secondary to previous cardiac interventions or the presence of pulmonary hypertension. In contrast to aortic regurgitation, pulmonary regurgitation better tolerated. However, in patients with free pulmonary regurgitation resulting in severe right ventricular dilatation, pulmonary valve replacement is required.

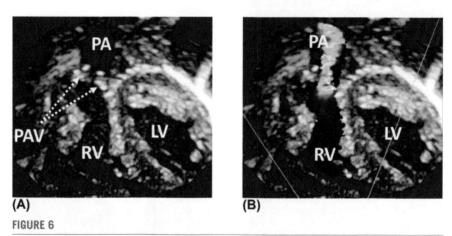

(A)   (B)

FIGURE 6

(A) Valvar pulmonary stenosis seen from the subcostal short-axis view. The pulmonary valve is severely dysplastic and thickened. Due to commissural fusion, the systolic opening of the valve is restricted, creating a "doming" appearance. (B) Color flow mapping showing turbulent flow across the valve. *LV,* left ventricle; *PA,* pulmonary artery; *PAV,* pulmonary valve; *RV,* right ventricle.

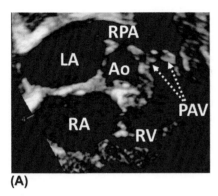
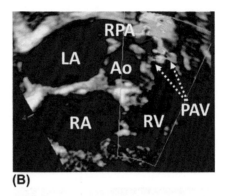

(A)   **(B)**

FIGURE 7

(A) Severe valvar pulmonary stenosis demonstrated from the subcostal short-axis view. The leaflets are very thickened and barely open in systole (doming). Note the poststenotic dilatation of the pulmonary artery. (B) Color flow mapping illustrating significantly reduced flow across the pulmonary valve. *Ao*, aorta; *LA*, left atrium; *LPA*, left pulmonary artery; *PAV*, pulmonary valve; *RA*, right atrium; *RLA*, right pulmonary artery; *RV*, right ventricle.

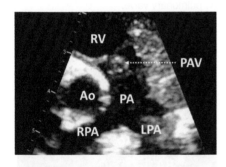

FIGURE 8

Zoomed parasternal short-axis view in a child with valvar pulmonary stenosis showing dysplasia and thickening of the leaflets. *Ao*, aorta; *LPA*, left pulmonary artery; *PA*, pulmonary artery; *PAV*, pulmonary valve; *RPA*, right pulmonary artery; *RV*, right ventricle.

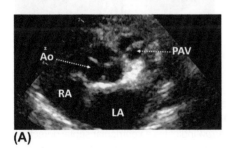
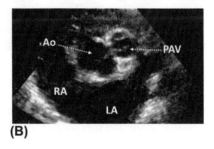

(A)   **(B)**

FIGURE 9

(A) High parasternal short-axis view demonstrating diastolic closure of a bicommissural (bicuspid) pulmonary valve in a child with pulmonary stenosis. There is hypoplasia of the pulmonary annulus. (B) Systolic opening of the valve. *Ao*, aorta; *LA*, left atrium; *PAV*, pulmonary valve; *RA*, right atrium.

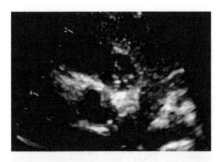

FIGURE 10

Severely dysplastic, tricommissural (tricuspid) pulmonary valve seen from the high parasternal short-axis view. There are commissural fusion and thickening of the leaflets. *Ao*, aorta; *LA*, left atrium; *PAV*, pulmonary valve.

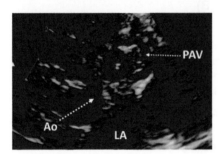

FIGURE 11

High parasternal short-axis view demonstrating a rare example of a quadricommissural (quadricuspid) pulmonary valve. There is a significant thickening of the leaflets, resulting in severe stenosis. *Ao*, aorta; *LA*, left atrium; *PAV*, pulmonary valve.

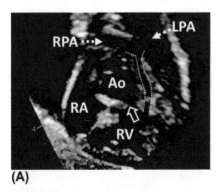 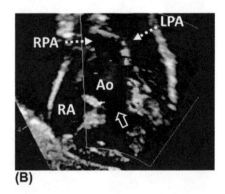

(A) **(B)**

FIGURE 12

(A) Subcostal short-axis view in a patient with tetralogy of Fallot and severe hypoplasia of the entire right ventricular outflow tract (RVOT) (*dotted lines*), resulting in obstruction at subvalvar, valvar, and supravalvar level. *Hollow arrow* indicates a ventricular septal defect (VSD). (B) Color flow mapping demonstrating turbulent flow across the RVOT. Due to the presence of severe RVOT obstruction, there is a right-to-left shunt across the VSD (*hollow arrow*). *Ao*, aorta; *LPA*, left pulmonary artery; *RA*, right atrium; *RPA*, right pulmonary artery; *RV*, right ventricle.

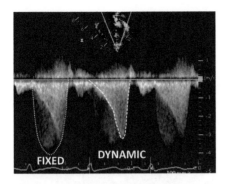

FIGURE 13

Continuous-wave Doppler of the right ventricular outflow tract (RVOT) in a patient with tetralogy of Fallot and multilevel obstruction. The triangular flow velocity waveform (*dashed line*) corresponds to the dynamic (subvalvar) component, which peaks toward the end of systole (when the contraction of the infundibulum reaches its maximum). The fixed (valvar or supravalvar) component has a rounded flow velocity waveform with a mid-systolic peak (*dotted line*).

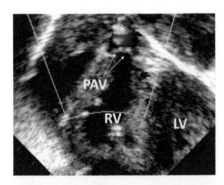

FIGURE 14

Subcostal short-axis view illustrating valvar pulmonary atresia. Note the absence of antegrade flow across the valve on color flow mapping. The flow in the pulmonary artery (asterisk) corresponds to ductal flow. *LV*, left ventricle; *PAV*, pulmonary valve; *RV*, right ventricle.

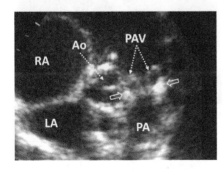

FIGURE 15

Parasternal short-axis view demonstrating valvar and supravalvar pulmonary stenosis in a child with geleophysic dysplasia. *Arrows* indicate the supravalvar component. *Ao*, aorta; *LA*, left atrium; *PA*, pulmonary artery; *PAV*, pulmonary valve; *RA*, right atrium.

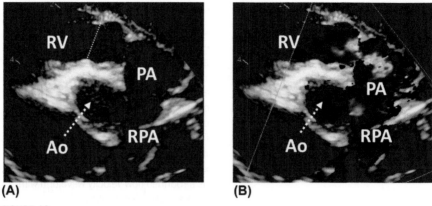

(A)   **(B)**

FIGURE 16

(A) Parasternal short-axis view in a child with significant supravalvar pulmonary stenosis. The *dotted line* represents the level of the pulmonary annulus. Note the poststenotic dilatation of the pulmonary artery. (B) Color flow mapping illustrating turbulent flow caused by the supravalvar obstruction. *Ao*, aorta; *PA*, pulmonary artery; *RPA*, right pulmonary artery; *RV*, right ventricle.

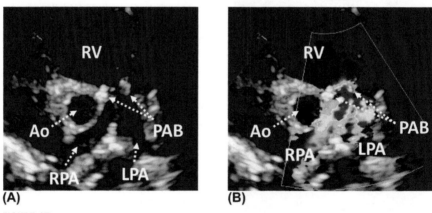

(A)   **(B)**

FIGURE 17

(A) In some patients with excessive pulmonary blood flow due to a shunt, pulmonary artery banding is performed to protect the pulmonary vascular bed. Parasternal short-axis view demonstrating a band that reduces the luminal diameter of the pulmonary artery (equivalent to supravalvar pulmonary stenosis). (B) Turbulent flow across the band on color flow mapping. *Ao*, aorta; *LPA*, left pulmonary artery; *PAB*, pulmonary artery band; *RPA*, right pulmonary artery; *RV*, right ventricle.

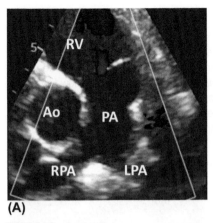

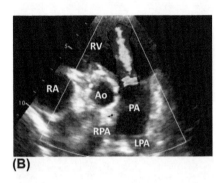

(A)   **(B)**

FIGURE 18

(A) Trivial (physiological) pulmonary regurgitation seen from the parasternal short-axis view. (B) Moderate pulmonary regurgitation in a patient with pulmonary hypertension. *Ao,* aorta; *LPA,* left pulmonary artery; *PAB,* pulmonary artery band; *RPA,* right pulmonary artery; *RV,* right ventricle.

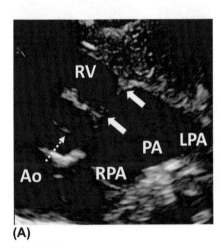

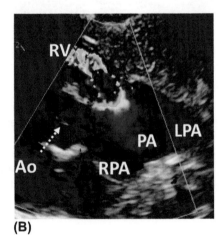

(A)   **(B)**

FIGURE 19

(A) Tetralogy of Fallot with absent pulmonary valve seen from a zoomed parasternal short-axis view. *Arrows* indicate the remnants of the valve. Note the severe dilatation of the pulmonary artery and its branches, which is a hallmark of the disease. (B) Free pulmonary regurgitation across the underdeveloped pulmonary valve. *Ao,* aorta; *LPA,* left pulmonary artery; *PA,* pulmonary artery; *RPA,* right pulmonary artery; *RV,* right ventricle.

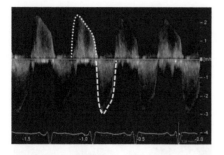

FIGURE 20

Same patient as in Figure 19. Continuous-wave Doppler of the right ventricular outflow tract showing both antegrade (*dashed line*) and retrograde flow (*dotted line*). The retrograde flow corresponds to free pulmonary regurgitation across the remnants of the valve.

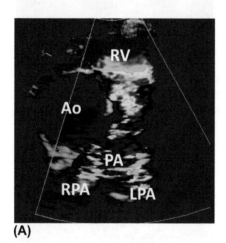

(A)

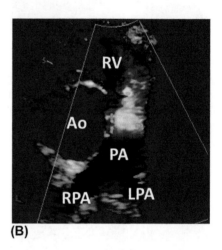

(B)

FIGURE 21

(A) Zoomed parasternal short-axis view demonstrating the right ventricular outflow tract (RVOT) in a patient with previous surgical repair of tetralogy of Fallot using a transannular patch. Color flow mapping showing mild residual flow turbulence across the RVOT. (B) Free pulmonary regurgitation caused by the presence of the patch. The regurgitant flow originates from the branch pulmonary arteries. *Ao*, aorta; *LPA*, left pulmonary artery; *PA*, pulmonary artery; *RPA*, right pulmonary artery; *RV*, right ventricle.

Double outlet right ventricle (DORV)

10

The term double outlet right ventricle (DORV) refers to a variety of cardiac defects, in which **both great arteries are connected by more than 50% to the right ventricle**. In DORV, both arterial valves are often separated from the atrio-ventricular valves by a sleeve of myocardium called the conus. However, the presence of a bilateral conus is not a determining factor of DORV. This is because in many patients with DORV and both great arteries committed predominantly to the right ventricle, only the subpulmonary conus exists, while the subaortic conus is absent (as in a normal heart where the aortic and mitral valves are in fibrous continuity).

It is important to mention that in a heart with a subaortic ventricular septal defect (VSD) and the aorta committed exclusively to the left ventricle, complete subpulmonary and subaortic conus with aorto-mitral discontinuity may exist. However, this abnormality cannot be labeled as DORV.

The **spatial relationship between the aorta and the pulmonary artery** is often **normal**. Nevertheless, **right anterior** or **left anterior** position of the aorta compared to the pulmonary artery or **side-by-side** arrangement of the great vessels is also possible. Another important feature used in describing DORV is the anatomical location and the commitment of the VSD to the valves of the great arteries. Based on this, we distinguish **DORV with subaortic, subpulmonary, doubly committed,** and **noncommitted VSD** (Figure 1).

The presence of subvalvar or valvar stenosis represents another factor that determines the resulting hemodynamic picture in patients with DORV. The subvalvar component of the outflow tract obstruction is usually caused by deviation of the infundibular septum against the ventricular free wall. Cardiac surgery is the only treatment in this heterogenous group of defects.

Atlas of Pediatric Echocardiography. https://doi.org/10.1016/B978-0-323-75981-6.00015-7

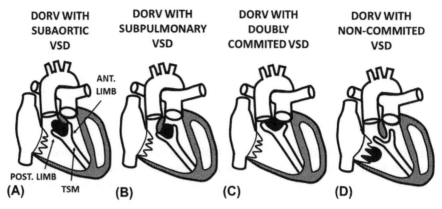

FIGURE 1

Classification of DORV based on the commitment of the ventricular septal defect (VSD) to the arterial valves. The infundibular septum (IS) is highlighted in brown. (A) In DORV with subaortic VSD, the IS fuses with the anterior limb of the septomarginal trabecula, which forms the left margin of the defect. (B) Fusion of the IS with the posterior limb of the septomarginal trabecula commits the VSD to the pulmonary valve. (C) DORV with doubly committed VSD is characterized by absent IS and commitment of the VSD to both arterial valves. (D) In DORV with noncommitted (remote) VSD, there is no alignment between the defect and the arterial valves. *ANT. LIMB*, anterior limb of TSM; *POST. LIMB*, postlimb of TSM; *TSM*, septomarginal trabecula.

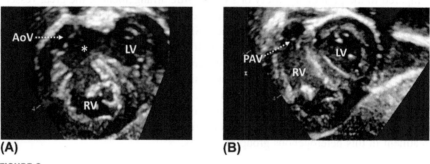

FIGURE 2

(A) Subcostal short-axis view in a child with DORV, normally related great arteries and subaortic ventricular septal defect (*asterisk*). The aortic valve is committed more to the right than to the left ventricle and overrides the interventricular septum. (B) Same heart seen from a more apical view. Note the origin of the pulmonary artery from the right ventricle. *AoV*, aortic valve; *LV*, left ventricle; *PAV*, pulmonary valve; *RV*, right ventricle.

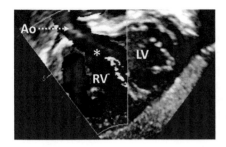

FIGURE 3

DORV with normally related great arteries and subaortic ventricular septal defect (*asterisk*) seen from the subcostal short-axis view. The aorta is committed more to the right than to the left ventricle and overrides the interventricular septum. Note the right-to-left shunt across the ventricular septal defect. *Ao*, aorta; *LV*, left ventricle; *RV*, right ventricle.

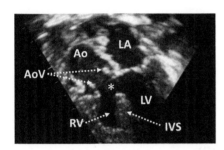

FIGURE 4

Apical five-chamber view illustrating the origin of the aorta from the right ventricle. The *asterisk* indicates a subaortic VSD. *Ao*, aorta; *AoV*, aortic valve; *IVS*, interventricular septum; *LA*, left atrium; *LV*, left ventricle; *RV*, right ventricle.

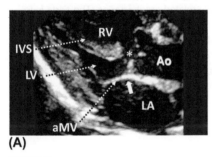

(A)

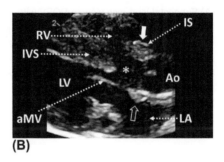

(B)

FIGURE 5

Parasternal long-axis view. (A) Patient with tetralogy of Fallot and 50% override of the aorta. Note the absence of subaortic conus, resulting in aortomitral continuity (*arrow*). The *asterisk* denotes a ventricular septal defect (VSD). (B) DORV with normally related great arteries, pulmonary stenosis (not shown), and subaortic VSD (*asterisk*). The *black and white arrows* indicate the subaortic conus, with the *black arrow* showing the separation of the aortic valve from the anterior mitral valve leaflet. *aMV*, anterior mitral valve leaflet; *Ao*, aorta; *IS*, infundibular septum; *IVS*, interventricular septum; *LA*, left atrium; *LV*, left ventricle; *RV*, right ventricle.

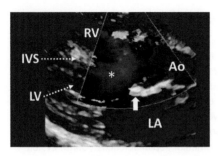

FIGURE 6

Parasternal long-axis view demonstrating >50% commitment of the aortic valve to the right ventricle. Color flow mapping illustrating a left-to-right shunt across the VSD (*asterisk*). *Ao,* aorta; *IVS,* interventricular septum; *LA,* left atrium; *LV,* left ventricle; *RV,* right ventricle.

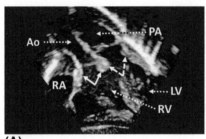

(A)

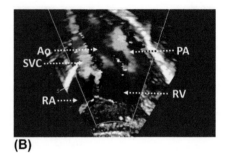

(B)

FIGURE 7

(A) Subcostal long-axis view in DORV with normally related great arteries. The aorta is to the right of the pulmonary artery. Note the presence of a double conus, with the plain *white arrows* indicating the subaortic conus and the *dashed white arrows* the subpulmonary conus. (B) Blood flow across both outflow tracts as demonstrated on color flow mapping. *Ao,* aorta; *LV,* left ventricle; *PA,* pulmonary artery; *RA,* right atrium; *RV,* right ventricle; *SVC,* superior vena cava.

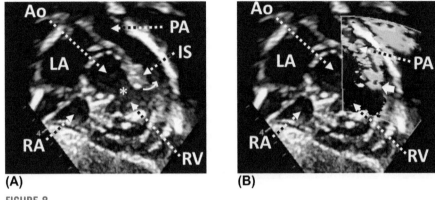

FIGURE 8

(A) Tetralogy of Fallot type DORV seen from the subcostal short-axis view. The *asterisk* indicates a subaortic ventricular septal defect. Note the hypertrophy and anterior deviation (*curved arrow*) of the infundibular septum, which is protruding into the right ventricular outflow tract (RVOT), causing its obstruction. (B) As a result, there is turbulent flow across the RVOT, starting at the level of the deviated infundibular septum (*arrow*). *Ao*, aorta; *IS*, infundibular septum; *LA*, left atrium; *PA*, pulmonary artery; *RA*, right atrium; *RV*, right ventricle.

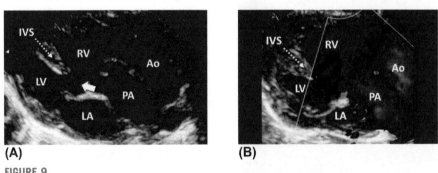

FIGURE 9

(A) Parasternal long-axis view illustrating transposition type DORV with right anterior aorta and subpulmonary ventricular septal defect (*arrow*). Note the double-barrel shotgun appearance of the great arteries. (B) There is a left-to-right shunt across the VSD as demonstrated on color flow mapping. The flow across the great arteries is unobstructed. *Ao*, aorta; *IVS*, interventricular septum; *LA*, left atrium; *LV*, left ventricle; *PA*, pulmonary artery; *RV*, right ventricle.

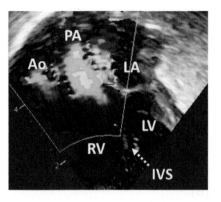

FIGURE 10

Transposition type DORV with side-by-side great arteries and subpulmonary VSD seen from the apical five-chamber view. The pulmonary artery is committed by >50% to the right ventricle. The aorta arises entirely from the right ventricle. *Ao*, aorta; *IVS*, interventricular septum; *LA*, left atrium; *LV*, left ventricle; *PA*, pulmonary artery; *RV*, right ventricle.

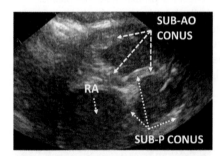

FIGURE 11

Zoomed high parasternal short-axis view in a child with transposition type DORV and right anterior aorta. Note the presence of a double conus. *Dashed arrows* indicate the subaortic conus and *dotted arrows* the subpulmonary conus. *RA*, right atrium; *SUB-AO CONUS subaortic conus, SUB-P CONUS subpulmonary conus.*

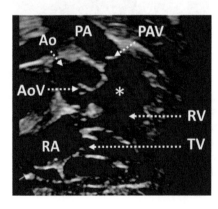

FIGURE 12

Subcostal short-axis view illustrating DORV with doubly committed ventricular septal defect (*asterisk*). Note the absence of the infundibular septum. The pulmonary valve is mildly hypoplastic in this patient. *Ao*, aorta; *AoV*, aortic valve; *PA*, pulmonary artery; *PAV*, pulmonary valve; *RA*, right atrium; *RV*, right ventricle; *TV*, tricuspid valve.

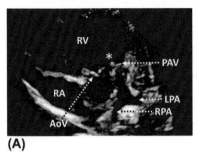 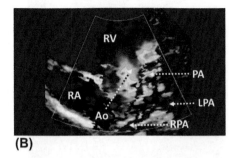

(A) **(B)**

FIGURE 13

(A) DORV with a doubly committed ventricular septal defect and pulmonary stenosis demonstrated from the parasternal short-axis view. There is an absence of the infundibular septum (*asterisk* indicates its usual position). (B) Color flow mapping showing blood flow in the aorta and the stenotic pulmonary artery. *AoV*, aortic valve; *LPA*, left pulmonary artery; *PA*, pulmonary artery; *PAV*, pulmonary valve; *RA*, right atrium; *RPA*, right pulmonary artery; *RV*, right ventricle.

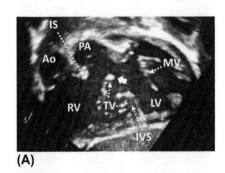 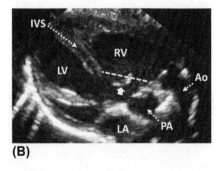

(A) **(B)**

FIGURE 14

(A) Subcostal short-axis view in a child with transposition type DORV (aorta to the right). There is a large inlet ventricular septal defect (VSD) with outlet extension. The VSD is noncommitted, that is, distant from both semilunar valves. The *arrow* indicates the marginal overriding of tricuspid valve tissue over the interventricular septum. (B) Same heart seen from a modified parasternal long-axis view. Note the protrusion of tricuspid valve tissue (*arrow*) into a hypothetical patch (*dashed line*) reconnecting the left ventricle to the neo-aorta after an arterial switch operation. This makes surgical repair difficult. *Ao*, aorta; *IS*, infundibular septum; *IVS*, interventricular septum; *LV*, left ventricle; *MV*, mitral valve; *PA*, pulmonary artery; *RV*, right ventricle; *TV*, tricuspid valve.

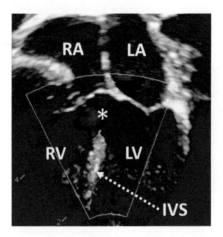

FIGURE 15

DORV with a large (noncommitted) inlet ventricular septal defect (*asterisk*) seen from the apical four-chamber view. Color flow mapping demonstrating a left-to-right shunt across the defect. Outflow tracts are not shown in this figure. *IVS*, interventricular septum; *LA*, left atrium; *LV*, left ventricle; *RA*, right atrium; *RV*, right ventricle.

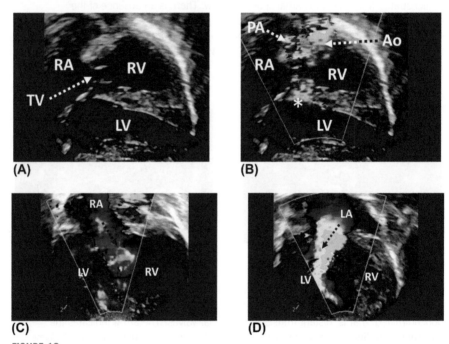

FIGURE 16

(A) Subcostal short-axis view showing a rare example of DORV with left anterior aorta and severe pulmonary stenosis. The inflow tracts have a criss-cross arrangement, resulting in a superior—inferior relationship of the atrio-ventricular (AV) valves and the ventricles. The tricuspid valve and the right ventricle (RV) lie superior to the mitral valve (not shown) and the left ventricle (LV). The interventricular septum is horizontal instead of being vertical. (B) The inferior LV is connected to the base of the RV via a large, inlet ventricular septal defect (*asterisk*). Both great arteries arise from the RV, with the aorta being to the left of the pulmonary artery. (C) Due to the superior—inferior relationship of the AV valves, it is not possible to simultaneously visualize the flow across both AV valves from the apical four-chamber view. The right-sided right atrium connects to a superiorly positioned left-sided RV. (D) The left-sided left atrium connects to an inferiorly positioned right-sided LV. *Ao*, aorta; *LA*, left atrium; *LV*, left ventricle; *LV*, left ventricle; *PA*, pulmonary artery; *RA*, right atrium; *RA* right atrium; *RV*, right ventricle; *RV*, right ventricle; *TV*, tricuspid valve.

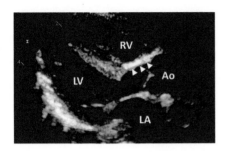

FIGURE 17

Parasternal long-axis view in a patient with tetralogy of Fallot-type DORV after full surgical repair. Arrowheads indicate the pericardial patch closing the ventricular septal defect and reconnecting the left ventricle to the aorta. *Ao,* aorta; *LA,* left atrium; *LV,* left ventricle; *RV,* right ventricle.

Tetralogy of Fallot

11

Tetralogy of Fallot is a complex cardiac malformation characterized by the presence of a multilevel right ventricular outflow tract obstruction, leading to right ventricular hypertrophy, and a malalignment ventricular septal defect with aortic override. The pulmonary valve is usually small and dysplastic, as is the pulmonary artery. In the **tetralogy of Fallot with pulmonary atresia**, which represents the extreme form of tetralogy of Fallot, the pulmonary valve is atretic.

Tetralogy of Fallot with absent pulmonary valve is a rare variant of the disease, where only nonfunctional remnants of the pulmonary valve are present. The characteristic feature of this condition is a strong dilatation of the pulmonary artery and its branches, causing airway compression.

Tetralogy of Fallot

The hemodynamic picture in the tetralogy of Fallot depends on the severity of pulmonary stenosis. In patients with mild obstruction, there is a left-to-right shunt across the ventricular septal defect, resulting in high oxygen saturations and clinical signs of high pulmonary blood flow. On the other hand, children with significant right ventricular outflow tract obstruction have a right-to-left shunt at the ventricular level and are cyanotic.

Right ventricular outflow tract obstruction can be at all three levels. Typically, the subvalvar component is due to an abnormal position of the infundibular septum, which protrudes into the subpulmonary infundibulum. Cyanotic spells, which develop in some patients, represent clinical equivalents of severe infundibular spasms. Valvar pulmonary stenosis is almost invariably present and is usually associated with obstruction at supravalvar level.

A number of palliative procedures can be performed in severely cyanotic patients as a bridge to surgical repair, with stenting of the right ventricular outflow tract being most often carried out. The vast majority of patients develop free pulmonary regurgitation after corrective surgery, leading to progressive right ventricular dilatation and the need for pulmonary valve replacement.

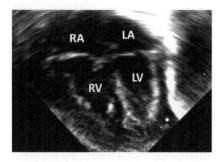

FIGURE 1

Apical four-chamber view showing significant right ventricular hypertrophy in a patient with tetralogy of Fallot and severe right ventricular outflow tract obstruction. *LA*, left atrium; *LV*, left ventricle; *RA*, right atrium; *RV*, right ventricle.

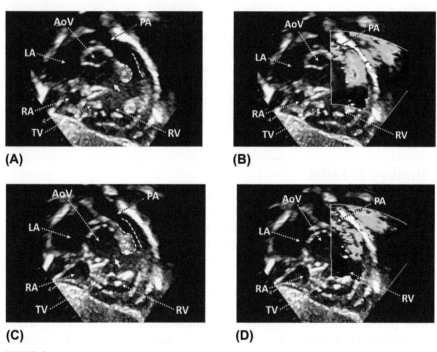

(A) **(B)**

(C) **(D)**

FIGURE 2

Subcostal short-axis view in a child with tetralogy of Fallot demonstrating dynamic changes in the severity of subvalvar pulmonary stenosis during systole. (A) The *asterisk* indicates the infundibular septum, which is hypertrophied and anteriorly deviated. The *arrow* denotes the ventricular septal defect. Early in systole, the space between the infundibular septum and the infundibular free wall (outlined by *dashed lines*) is relatively wide. (B) The flow across the subpulmonary infundibulum is only mildly turbulent due to the protrusion of the infundibular septum into it. (C) Toward the end of systole, when the infundibular myocardium is maximally contracted, the space outlined by the *dashed lines* becomes very narrow. (D) Resulting severe subvalvar pulmonary stenosis, as demonstrated on color flow mapping. *AoV*, aortic valve; *PA*, pulmonary artery; *RV*, right ventricle; *TV*, tricuspid valve.

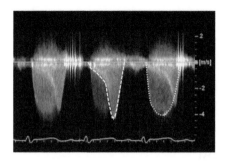

FIGURE 3

Continuous-wave Doppler of the right ventricular outflow tract in a patient with tetralogy of Fallot. The dynamic obstruction caused by the contraction of the infundibulum has a triangular flow velocity waveform (*dashed line*) and peaks toward the end of systole. The fixed (valvar and supravalvar) component does not progress in systole and has a rounded flow velocity waveform with a mid-systolic peak (*dotted line*). Both waveforms are superimposed.

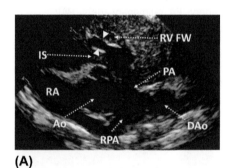

(A)

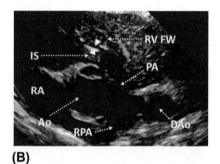

(B)

FIGURE 4

(A) Parasternal short-axis view in a patient with tetralogy of Fallot and frequent cyanotic spells. *Arrowheads* indicate the lumen of the subpulmonary infundibulum in early systole. (B) Note the almost complete collapse of the infundibulum at the end of systole (*arrowheads*). *Ao,* aorta; *DAo,* descending aorta; *IS,* infundibular septum; *PA,* pulmonary artery; *RA,* right atrium; *RPA,* right pulmonary artery; *RV FW,* free wall of the subpulmonary infdundibulum.

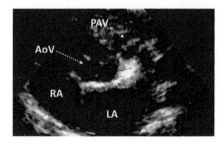

FIGURE 5

Parasternal short-axis view showing a bicommissural (bicuspid) pulmonary valve in a child with tetralogy of Fallot and valvar pulmonary stenosis. There is a hypoplasia of the pulmonary annulus. *AoV,* aortic valve; *LA,* left atrium; *PAV,* pulmonary valve; *RA,* right atrium.

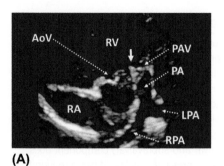 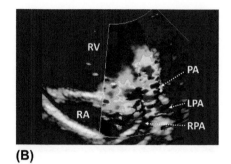

(A) **(B)**

FIGURE 6

(A) Parasternal short-axis view in a child with tetralogy of Fallot with doubly committed ventricular septal defect. The *arrow* indicates the absence of the infundibular septum. (B) Turbulent flow across the right ventricular outflow tract as demonstrated on color flow mapping. *AoV*, aortic valve; *LPA*, left pulmonary artery; *PA*, pulmonary artery; *PAV*, pulmonary valve; *RA*, right atrium; *RPA*, right pulmonary artery; *RV*, right ventricle.

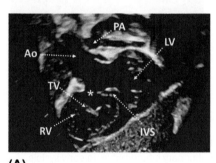 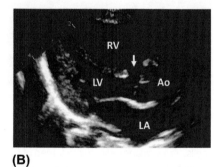

(A) **(B)**

FIGURE 7

(A) Subcostal five-chamber view demonstrating an overriding aorta in a patient with tetralogy of Fallot. The *asterisk* indicates subaortic ventricular septal defect. (B) Parasternal long-axis view illustrating an overriding aorta with less than 50% commitment of the aortic valve to the right ventricle. The *arrow* denotes the ventricular septal defect. *Ao*, aorta; *IVS*, interventricular septum; *LA*, left atrium; *LV*, left ventricle; *PA*, pulmonary artery; *RV*, right ventricle; *TV*, tricuspid valve.

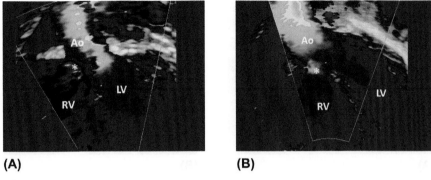

(A)   (B)

FIGURE 8

(A) Apical five-chamber view demonstrating a systolic left-to-right shunt across the ventricular septal defect (VSD) (*asterisk*) in a child with tetralogy of Fallot and mild right ventricular outflow tract obstruction. (B) Different patient with tight pulmonary stenosis and a systolic right-to- left shunt across the VSD (*asterisk*). Note the overriding aorta is dilated. *Ao*, aorta; *LV*, left ventricle; *RV*, right ventricle.

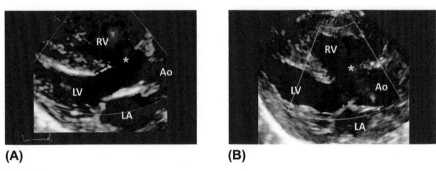

(A)   (B)

FIGURE 9

(A) Parasternal long axis view in a child with "pink" tetralogy of Fallot and mild pulmonary stenosis. There is a left-to-right shunt across the ventricular septal defect (VSD) (*asterisk*) due to a mild degree of pulmonary stenosis. Note the overriding aorta. (B) Right-to-left shunt across the VSD (*asterisk*) in a patient with significant right ventricular outflow tract obstruction. *Ao*, aorta; *LV*, left ventricle; *MV*, mitral valve; *RV*, right ventricle.

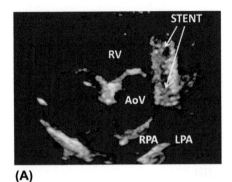
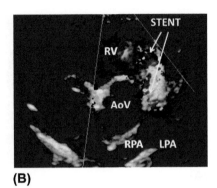

(A) **(B)**

FIGURE 10

(A) Preterm infant with tetralogy of Fallot and frequent cyanotic spells who required stenting of the right ventricular outflow tract as a bridge to surgical repair. The stent covers the full length of the infundibulum. (B) Color flow mapping demonstrating retrograde (regurgitant) diastolic flow across the stent. *AoV*, aortic valve; *LPA*, left pulmonary artery; *RPA*, right pulmonary artery; *RV*, right ventricle.

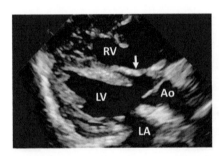

FIGURE 11

Parasternal long-axis view in a patient with tetralogy of Fallot after complete surgical repair. The *arrow* indicates patch closure of the ventricular septal defect. *Ao*, aorta; *LA*, left atrium; *LV*, left ventricle; *RV*, right ventricle.

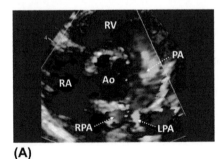
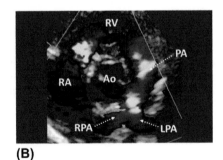

(A) **(B)**

FIGURE 12

(A) Patient with tetralogy of Fallot who underwent complete surgical repair with transannular patch. The *asterisk* indicates a patch closing the subaortic ventricular septal defect. Color flow mapping demonstrating laminar flow across the right ventricular outflow tract. (B) Residual free pulmonary regurgitation originating from the branch pulmonary arteries and meeting with the tricuspid inflow. *Ao*, aorta; *LPA*, left pulmonary artery; *PA*, pulmonary artery; *RA*, right atrium; *RPA*, right pulmonary artery; *RV*, right ventricle.

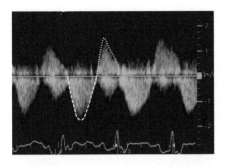

FIGURE 13

Same patient as in Figure 11. Continuous-wave Doppler of the right ventricular outflow tract showing both antegrade (*dashed line*) and regurgitant flow (*dotted line*).

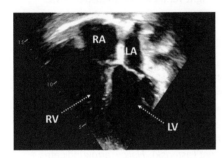

FIGURE 14

Patient with tetralogy of Fallot several years after surgical repair with transannular patch. Note the severe right ventricular dilatation caused by residual free pulmonary regurgitation. *LA*, left atrium; *LV*, left ventricle; *RA*, right atrium; *RV*, right ventricle.

Tetralogy of Fallot with pulmonary atresia

In the tetralogy of Fallot with pulmonary atresia, no flow can be detected from the right ventricle to the pulmonary artery. This is usually caused by muscular obliteration of the infundibulum and less often by membranous atresia of the valve. The pulmonary artery is usually hypoplastic. The branch pulmonary arteries are well developed and confluent at one end of the spectrum and hypoplastic or even absent on the other. In the latter case, the pulmonary blood supply depends on blood flow from major aorto-pulmonary collaterals (MAPCAs).

The initial palliation in patients with tetralogy of Fallot with pulmonary atresia consists either in the creation of a surgical shunt, arterial duct stenting, or right ventricular outflow tract augmentation (surgical or percutaneous). In many of these children, a more definitive long-term treatment is often very difficult.

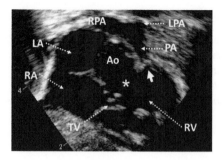

FIGURE 15

Tetralogy of Fallot with pulmonary atresia demonstrated from the subcostal short-axis view. The *arrow* indicates an atretic pulmonary valve. Note the severe hypoplasia of the pulmonary artery and its branches. The *asterisk* denotes a large ventricular septal defect. *Ao*, aorta; *LA*, left atrium; *LPA*, left pulmonary artery; *RA*, right atrium; *RPA*, right pulmonary artery; *RV*, right ventricle; *TV*, tricuspid valve.

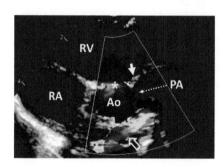

FIGURE 16

Parasternal short-axis view in a child with tetralogy of Fallot with pulmonary atresia. The *arrow* indicates the muscular obliteration of the infundibulum. Color flow mapping showing an obligatory right-to-left shunt across the ventricular septal defect (*asterisk*). *Hollow arrow* indicates a major aorto-pulmonary collateral contributing to pulmonary blood flow. *Ao*, aorta; *PA*, pulmonary artery; *RA*, right atrium; *RPA*, right pulmonary artery; *RV*, right ventricle.

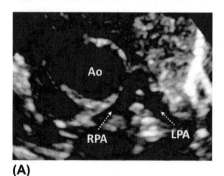

(A)

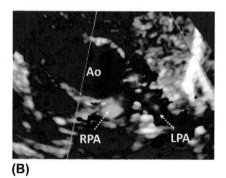

(B)

FIGURE 17

(A) Zoomed left subclavicular view in a patient with tetralogy of Fallot with pulmonary atresia. The branch pulmonary arteries are confluent and severely hypoplastic. (B) Color flow mapping demonstrating blood flow in the branch pulmonary arteries. *Ao*, aorta; *LPA*, left pulmonary artery; *RPA*, right pulmonary artery.

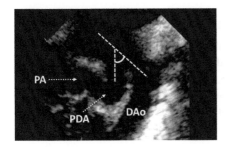

FIGURE 18

Suprasternal notch view in a newborn with tetralogy of Fallot with pulmonary atresia. In malformations with significantly reduced or no antegrade flow across the pulmonary valve in utero, the lungs are supplied retrogradely from the aorta. This results in the reverse orientation of the duct (sharp angle) as illustrated in this example. *DAo*, descending aorta; *PA*, pulmonary artery; *PDA*, patent ductus arteriosus.

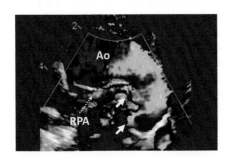

FIGURE 19

Tetralogy of Fallot with pulmonary atresia and major aorto-pulmonary collaterals (MAPCAs) (*arrows*) visualized from the suprasternal notch view. Direct communication between one of the collaterals and the right pulmonary artery is shown. *Ao*, aorta; *RPA*, right pulmonary artery.

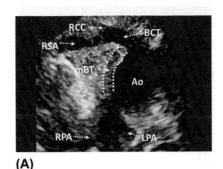

(A)

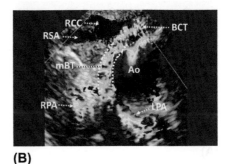

(B)

FIGURE 20

(A) Suprasternal notch view demonstrating the aortic origin of the brachiocephalic trunk in a child with tetralogy of Fallot with pulmonary atresia. Note the presence of a modified Blalock–Taussig shunt (*dashed lines*) originating from the base of the brachiocephalic trunk and connecting to the branch pulmonary arteries. (B) Color flow mapping showing turbulent flow across the shunt and the branch pulmonary arteries. *Ao*, aorta; *BCT*, braciocephalic trunk; *LPA*, left pulmonary artery; *mBT*, modified Blalock – Taussig shunt; *RCC*, right common carotid artery; *RPA*, right pulmonary artery; *RSA*, right subclavian artery.

Tetralogy of Fallot with absent pulmonary valve

Tetralogy of Fallot with absent pulmonary valve is characterized by the presence of a malformed, rudimentary pulmonary valve that is both stenotic and regurgitant. A key feature of this condition is the extreme dilatation of the pulmonary artery and its branches, which in some patients causes significant compression and underdevelopment of the airways. As in tetralogy of Fallot, there is a large malalignment ventricular septal defect.

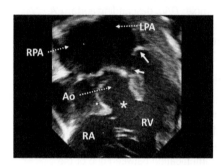

FIGURE 21

Subcostal short-axis view in an infant with tetralogy of Fallot with absent pulmonary valve, severe airway compression, and ventilator dependence. *Arrows* indicate the remnants of the pulmonary valve. Note the severe dilatation of the pulmonary artery and its branches. *Asterisk* denotes the ventricular septal defect. *Ao*, aorta; *LPA*, left pulmonary artery; *LV*, left ventricle; *RPA*, right pulmonary artery; *RV*, right ventricle; *RV*, right ventricle.

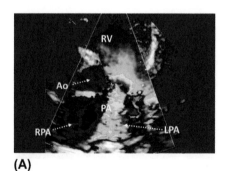

(A)

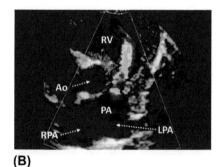

(B)

FIGURE 22

(A) Parasternal short-axis view in a child with tetralogy of Fallot with absent pulmonary valve. Color flow mapping demonstrating turbulent flow across the remnants of the valve. There is severe dilatation of the pulmonary artery and its branches, with swirling flow in the right pulmonary artery. (B) Free pulmonary regurgitation caused by the lack of a competent valve. *Ao*, aorta; *LPA*, left pulmonary artery; *PA*, pulmonary artery; *RPA*, right pulmonary artery; *RV*, right ventricle.

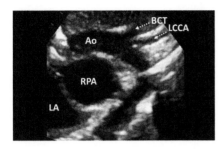

FIGURE 23

Suprasternal notch view demonstrating extreme dilatation of the right pulmonary artery in a patient with tetralogy of Fallot with absent pulmonary valve. *Ao*, aorta; *BCT*, brachiocephalic trunk; *LA*, left atrium; *LCCA*, left common carotid artery; *RPA*, right pulmonary artery.

Transposition of the great arteries (TGA)

12

Transposition of the great arteries (TGA) is a common congenital heart defect characterized by ventriculo-arterial discordance. In this condition, the aorta arises anteriorly from the morphological right ventricle and the pulmonary artery posteriorly from the morphological left ventricle. As a result, the circulatory system consists of two separate (parallel) circuits, with the oxygen-rich blood circulating in the pulmonary circuit and the deoxygenated blood in the systemic circuit.

Early survival in patients with TGA depends on the mixing of blood between the two circuits. This occurs at intracardiac level (atrial or ventricular septal defects) or at extracardiac level (patent arterial duct or bronchopulmonary collaterals). TGA is most often an isolated lesion, but it may also be associated with other cardiac anomalies, typically including ventricular septal defect and /or left ventricular outflow tract obstruction. Less commonly, ventriculo-arterial discordance is part of some more complex malformations.

Isolated TGA is a critical heart defect, which often requires balloon atrial septostomy in the early postnatal period. However, its use has decreased due to widespread availability of prostaglandins. In patients with TGA, ventriculo-arterial concordance can only be restored surgically. Detailed examination of the coronary artery anatomy, which plays an important role in the preparation for arterial switch operation, is described in Chapter 20.

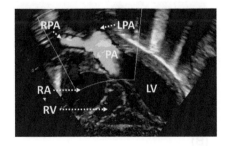

FIGURE 1

Subcostal long-axis view in a newborn with isolated TGA. Color flow mapping demonstrating the origin of the pulmonary artery from the left ventricle. *LPA*, left pulmonary artery; *LV*, left ventricle; *PA*, pulmonary artery; *RA*, right atrium; *RPA*, right pulmonary artery; *RV*, right ventricle.

Atlas of Pediatric Echocardiography. https://doi.org/10.1016/B978-0-323-75981-6.00016-9

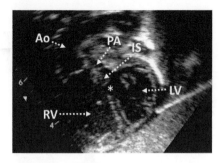

FIGURE 2

Patient with TGA, ventricular septal defect (*asterisk*), and subvalvar and valvar pulmonary stenosis. Subcostal five-chamber axis view illustrating the origin of the aorta from the right ventricle. The pulmonary artery is hypoplastic and arises from the left ventricle. The infundibular septum is hypertrophied and protrudes into the left ventricular outflow tract, causing its obstruction. *Ao*, aorta; *IS*, infundibular septum; *LV*, left ventricle; *PA*, pulmonary artery; *RV*, right ventricle.

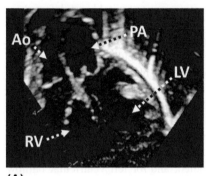

(A)

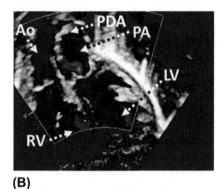

(B)

FIGURE 3

(A) TGA with intact interventricular septum seen from the subcostal five-chamber view. In contrast to a normal heart, where the outflow tracts and the great arteries are in a crossed relationship, they have a parallel orientation in TGA. The aorta is connected to the right ventricle and the pulmonary artery to the left ventricle. (B) Color flow mapping showing ductal flow to the pulmonary artery. *Ao*, aorta; *LV*, left ventricle; *PA*, pulmonary artery; *PDA*, patent ductus arteriosus; *RV*, right ventricle.

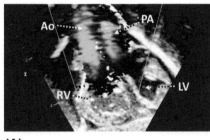

(A)

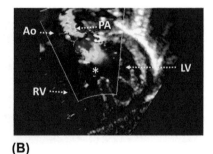

(B)

FIGURE 4

(A) Subcostal five-chamber view with color flow mapping illustrating the parallel course of both great arteries in an infant with isolated TGA. (B) Patient with TGA, large ventricular septal defect (*asterisk*), and valvar and subvalvar pulmonary stenosis. Both great arteries run parallel to each other. Note the turbulent flow across the left ventricular outflow tract and the pulmonary valve. *Ao*, aorta; *LV*, left ventricle; *PA*, pulmonary artery; *RV*, right ventricle.

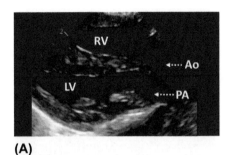
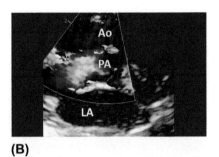

(A)   **(B)**

FIGURE 5

(A) Parasternal long-axis view in a newborn with isolated TGA. Note the parallel course of the great arteries creating an appearance of a double-barrel shotgun. (B) Color flow mapping showing blood flow across the aorta and the pulmonary artery. *Ao*, aorta; *LV*, left ventricle; *PA*, pulmonary artery; *RV*, right ventricle.

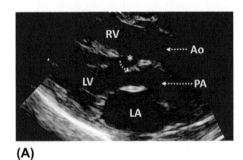
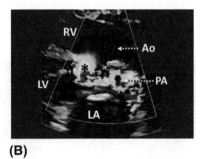

(A)   **(B)**

FIGURE 6

(A) Parasternal long-axis view in an infant with TGA, ventricular septal defect (*asterisk*), and subvalvar and valvar pulmonary stenosis. The infundibular septum is posteriorly deviated (*curved dotted arrow*), protruding into the left ventricular outflow tract. The caliber of the pulmonary artery is smaller than that of the aorta. (B) Color flow mapping demonstrating turbulent flow across the left ventricular outflow tract starting at the level of the deviated infundibular septum. The direction of the shunt across the ventricular septal defect (*asterisk*) is from the systemic right ventricle to the subpulmonary left ventricle. *Ao*, aorta; *LA*, left atrium; *LV*, left ventricle; *PA*, pulmonary artery; *RV*, right ventricle.

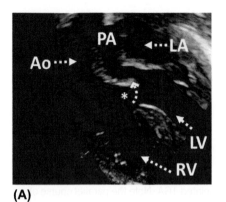 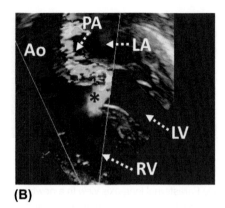

(A) **(B)**

FIGURE 7

(A) Same heart as in Figure 6 seen from the subcostal five-chamber view. *Asterisk* indicates the ventricular septal defect, *curved dotted arrow* the deviation of the infundibular septum. (B) Color flow mapping showing obstruction to the flow across the left ventricular outflow tract caused by the deviated infundibular septum. *Ao*, aorta; *LA*, left atrium; *LV*, left ventricle; *PA*, pulmonary artery; *RV*, right ventricle.

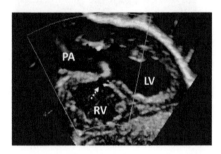

FIGURE 8

Subcostal short-axis view in a newborn with TGA, small ventricular septal defect (*dotted arrow*), and unobstructed left ventricular outflow tract. Note the right-to-left shunt across the defect (from the systemic right ventricle to the subpulmonary left ventricle). *LV*, left ventricle; *PA*, pulmonary artery; *RV*, right ventricle.

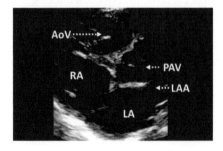

FIGURE 9

High parasternal short-axis view illustrating the spatial relationship of the great arteries in TGA. Note the right anterior position of the aorta compared to the pulmonary artery. *AoV*, aortic valve; *LA*, left atrium; *LAA*, left atrial appendage; *PAV*, pulmonary valve; *RA*, right atrium.

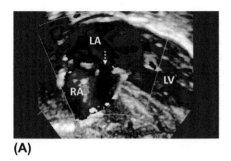
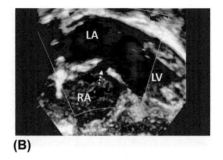

(A)   **(B)**

FIGURE 10

Subcostal four-chamber view illustrating mixing of blood at the atrial level in a newborn with TGA. There is bidirectional flow across a rather small atrial communication (*dotted arrow*) (A) Left-to-right shunt. (B) Right-to-left shunt. *LA*, left atrium; *LV*, left ventricle; *RA*, right atrium.

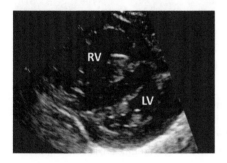

FIGURE 11

Detailed examination of the left ventricular (LV) geometry is important in patients with TGA and intact interventricular septum, whom the arterial switch operation is delayed and preoperative left ventricular deconditioning may have occurred due to the drop in pulmonary vascular resistance. Parasternal short-axis view in an infant with isolated TGA. The systemic right ventricle (RV) is dilated and has a rounded shape, while the subpulmonary left ventricle has a crescent-like appearance.

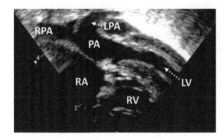

FIGURE 12

In isolated TGA, the shape of the left ventricle depends on the interventricular pressure ratio. Subcostal long-axis view demonstrating right ventricular dilatation and left ventricular compression caused by the right-to-left bowing of the interventricular septum. *LPA*, left pulmonary artery; *LV*, left ventricle; *PA*, pulmonary artery; *RA*, right atrium; *RPA*, right pulmonary artery; *RV*, right ventricle.

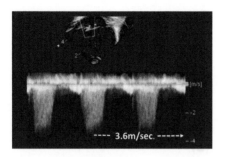

FIGURE 13

Continuous-wave Doppler of the tricuspid valve from the apical four-chamber view in a newborn with isolated TGA. The tricuspid regurgitation peak velocity is high (3.6 m/s in this example), due to systemic pressure in the right ventricle.

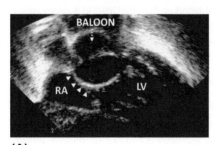

(A)

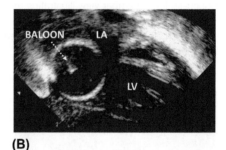

(B)

FIGURE 14

Balloon atrial septostomy is usually required in patients with isolated TGA, restrictive atrial septum, and poor atrial level mixing. (A) Subcostal four-chamber view demonstrating an inflated septostomy balloon in the left atrium. *Arrowheads* indicate the atrial septum. (B) After perforation of the atrial septum, the balloon is in the right atrium. *LA*, left atrium; *LV*, left ventricle; *RA*, right atrium.

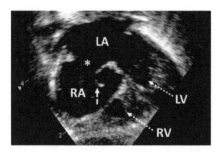

FIGURE 15

Large atrial communication (*asterisk*) seen from the subcostal four-chamber view in a newborn with isolated TGA who underwent balloon atrial septostomy. *Dashed arrow* indicates a flail remnant of torn septal tissue. *LA*, left atrium; *LV*, left ventricle; *RA*, right atrium; *RV*, right ventricle.

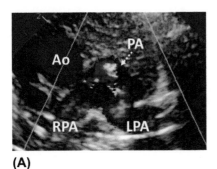 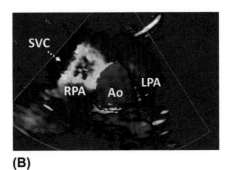

(A)   **(B)**

FIGURE 16

(A) Spatial relationship of the great arteries in a newborn with isolated TGA demonstrated from the left subclavicular view. Note the right-anterior position of the aorta compared to the bifurcating pulmonary artery. (B) Anteroposterior relationship of the great arteries after arterial switch operation. During this procedure, the ascending aorta was positioned behind the pulmonary artery bifurcation (Lecompte maneuver). *Ao*, aorta; *LPA*, left pulmonary artery; *RPA*, right pulmonary artery; *SVC*, superior vena cava.

Congenitally corrected transposition of the great arteries (CCTGA)

13

Congenitally corrected transposition of the great arteries (CCTGA) is a rare cardiac defect characterized by discordance at the atrio-ventricular and ventriculo-arterial level. This is due to an abnormal, leftward looping of the primitive heart tube in utero, resulting in the morphological right ventricle being on the left side of the morphological left ventricle. Because of the presence of double discordance, this defect is physiologically corrected while maintaining blood flow from the left atrium to the aorta and from the right atrium to the pulmonary artery.

CCTGA is frequently associated with the presence of dextrocardia, mesocardia, ventricular septal defects, pulmonary stenosis or atresia, and Ebsteinoid malformation of the tricuspid valve. Progressive tricuspid valve disease and systemic right ventricular failure are worrisome complications that contribute significantly to the morbidity and mortality of these patients. Conduction disorders on ECG represent another characteristic feature of this condition.

Associated cardiac defects usually require surgical repair in early life. Some patients with right ventricular failure and preserved left ventricular function may benefit from anatomical repair (double-switch operation) that is achieved by redirecting blood flow at the level of the atria and the great arteries. In some cases, pulmonary artery banding is required before the double-switch operation to "train" the morphological left ventricle to later become systemic.

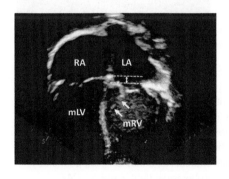

FIGURE 1

Apical four-chamber view in a patient with CCTGA demonstrating atrio-ventricular discordance. The *arrows* indicate attachment of the septal leaflet of the tricuspid valve to the interventricular septum. *Dashed lines* represent the mild apical displacement of the tricuspid valve in relation to the mitral valve. These features, among others, characterize the morphological right ventricle, which is on the left side of the heart in this child. *LA*, left atrium; *mLV*, morphological left ventricle; *mRV*, morphological right ventricle; *RA*, right atrium.

Atlas of Pediatric Echocardiography. https://doi.org/10.1016/B978-0-323-75981-6.00026-1

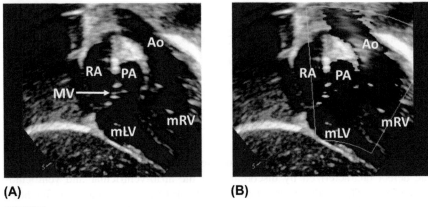

(A) (B)

FIGURE 2

(A) Subcostal long-axis view showing ventriculo-arterial discordance in CCTGA. The aorta arises anteriorly from the morphological right ventricle, which is coarsely trabeculated. The pulmonary artery is posterior to the aorta and originates from the morphological left ventricle, which has a smooth endocardial surface. Note the parallel orientation of the great arteries. (B) Corresponding color flow mapping in the same child. *Ao*, aorta; *mLV*, morphological left ventricle; *mRV*, morphological right ventricle; *MV*, mitral valve; *PA*, pulmonary artery; *RA*, right atrium.

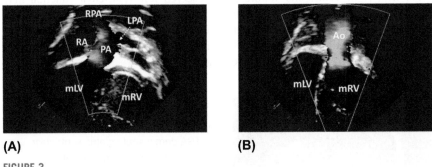

(A) (B)

FIGURE 3

(A) Apical five-chamber view demonstrating ventriculo-arterial discordance in a patient with CCTGA. Color flow mapping illustrating the origin of the pulmonary artery from the (right-sided) morphological left ventricle. (B) More anterior plane showing the origin of the aorta from the (left-sided) morphological right ventricle. The aorta is to the left of the pulmonary artery and both vessels have a parallel course. *Ao*, aorta; *LPA*, left pulmonary artery; *mLV*, morphological left ventricle; *mRV*, morphological right ventricle; *PA*, pulmonary artery; *RA*, right atrium; *RPA*, right pulmonary artery.

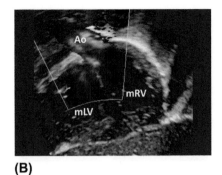

(A)   **(B)**

FIGURE 4

(A) Subcostal short-axis view demonstrating ventriculo-arterial discordance in a patient with CCTGA. The pulmonary artery arises from the (right-sided) morphological left ventricle. (B) The aorta is connected to the (left-sided) morphological right ventricle. The interventricular septum is intact. *Ao*, aorta; *mLV*, morphological left ventricle; *mRV*, morphological right ventricle; *PA*, pulmonary artery.

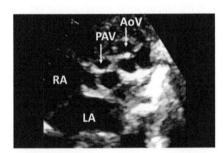

FIGURE 5

High parasternal short axis view demonstrating the spatial relationship of the aorta and the pulmonary artery in CCTGA. The aorta is anterior and to the left of the pulmonary artery. *AoV*, aortic valve; *LA*, left atrium; *PAV*, pulmonary artery valve; *RA*, right atrium.

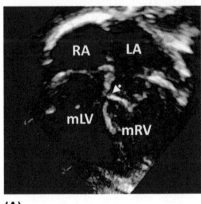
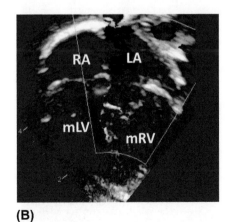

(A)   **(B)**

FIGURE 6

(A) Apical four-chamber view in a child with CCTGA and Ebsteinoid malformation of the tricuspid valve. Note the apical displacement of the septal leaflet hinge point (*arrow*). (B) Color flow mapping showing a trivial degree of tricuspid regurgitation. *LA*, left atrium; *mLV*, morphological left ventricle; *mRV*, morphological right ventricle; *RA*, right atrium.

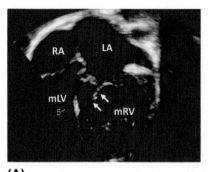

(A)

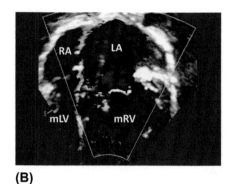

(B)

FIGURE 7

(A) Same patient as in Figure 6, seen 2 years later. Apical four-chamber view demonstrating significant dilatation of the left atrium and the morphological right ventricle caused by severe tricuspid regurgitation. The *arrows* indicate attachment of the septal leaflet of the tricuspid valve to the interventricular septum. (B) Color flow mapping illustrating significant progression of the tricuspid regurgitation compared to Figure 6B. Note the severe, eccentric regurgitant jet, extending deep into the left atrium. *LA,* left atrium; *mLV,* morphological left ventricle; *mRV,* morphological right ventricle; *RA,* right atrium.

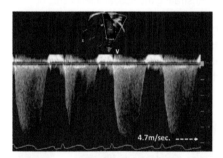

FIGURE 8

Continuous-wave Doppler of the tricuspid valve from the apical four-chamber view in a child with CCTGA. This figure shows the regurgitant signal only. The tricuspid regurgitation peak velocity is 4.7 m/s, which corresponds to the systemic pressure generated by the right ventricle.

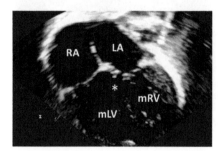

FIGURE 9

Apical four-chamber view in a patient with CCTGA and a large inlet ventricular septal defect (*asterisk*) with outlet extension. The tricuspid valve and the mitral valve are offset. *LA,* left atrium; *mLV,* morphological left ventricle; *mRV,* morphological right ventricle; *RA,* right atrium.

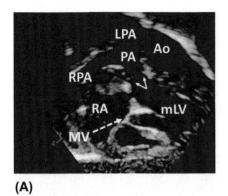
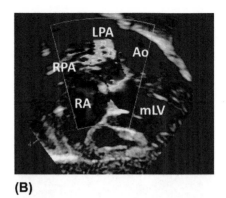

(A)   **(B)**

FIGURE 10

(A) Subcostal five-chamber view in a patient with CCTGA with valvar pulmonary stenosis. The pulmonary valve is thickened and doming (*arrows*). (B) Color flow mapping demonstrating turbulent flow across the valve. *Ao*, aorta; *LPA*, left pulmonary artery; *mLV*, morphological left ventricle; *MV*, mitral valve; *PA*, pulmonary artery; *RA*, right atrium; *RPA*, right pulmonary artery.

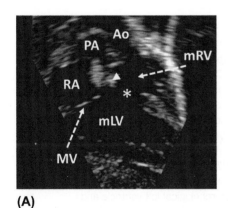
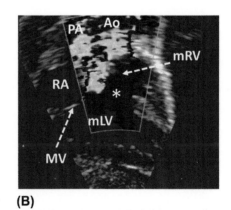

(A)   **(B)**

FIGURE 11

(A) Subcostal view in a child with CCTGA and an outlet ventricular septal defect (VSD) (*asterisk*). The *arrowhead* indicates deviation of the infundibular septum that protrudes into the left ventricular outflow tract (LVOT) causing severe subpulmonary stenosis. (B) Color flow mapping demonstrating turbulent flow across the LVOT starting at the level of the deviated infundibular septum. Due to the severity of the obstruction, the shunt across the VSD is from the morphological left to the morphological right ventricle. *Ao*, aorta; *mLV*, morphological left ventricle; *mRV*, morphological right ventricle; *MV*, mitral valve; *PA*, pulmonary artery; *RA*, right atrium.

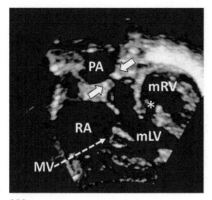
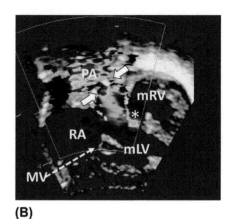

(A)   **(B)**

FIGURE 12

(A) Subcostal five-chamber view in a patient with CCTGA and a small ventricular septal defect (*asterisk*) who underwent pulmonary artery banding. *Arrows* indicate the luminal narrowing of the pulmonary artery caused by the band. (B) Color flow mapping illustrating turbulent flow across the band. The shunt across the ventricular septal defect is from the morphological right to the morphological left ventricle. *mLV*, morphological left ventricle; *mRV*, morphological right ventricle; *MV*, mitral valve; *PA*, pulmonary artery; *RA*, right atrium.

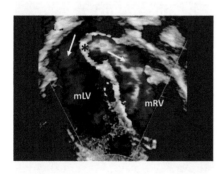

FIGURE 13

Apical four-chamber view in a child with CCTGA after the double-switch operation. The first part of this procedure consists in redirecting blood flow at the atrial level (Senning procedure), which is achieved by creating an interatrial baffle from autologous atrial tissue (*black asterisk*). *White arrows* indicate redirection of pulmonary venous return to the morphological left ventricle and redirection of the systemic venous return to the morphological right ventricle. The second part of the double-switch operation is the arterial switch procedure (see Chapter 12, Figure 16B). mRV morphological right ventricle, mLV morphological left ventricle.

Persistent truncus arteriosus

14

Persistent truncus arteriosus is a rare cardiac defect caused by the failure of the primitive arterial trunk to divide into the aorta and the pulmonary artery. Thus, the heart has a single outlet in the form of an arterial vessel supplying the systemic, pulmonary, and coronary circulation. The truncal valve is committed to both ventricles and overrides the outlet ventricular septal defect. Truncal valve dysplasia is frequently observed, resulting in varying degrees of stenosis and/or regurgitation. The number of cusps may also differ among patients, ranging from bicommissural (bicuspid) to hexacommissural (hexacuspid) valves.

Based on the origin of the branch pulmonary arteries, three different types of truncus arteriosus are distinguished. In **type I**, the truncus gives rise to the pulmonary artery, which then bifurcates into two branches. In **type II**, the right and left pulmonary arteries have close, but separate origins from the truncus. In **type III**, the origin of both pulmonary arteries is more distant.

Persistent truncus arteriosus is associated with interrupted aortic arch in approximately 15% of cases and in one-third of patients with DiGeorge syndrome. Infants with persistent truncus arteriosus typically develop early symptoms of heart failure and require corrective surgery in the first few weeks of life.

Atlas of Pediatric Echocardiography. https://doi.org/10.1016/B978-0-323-75981-6.00005-4

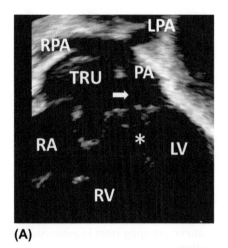

(A)

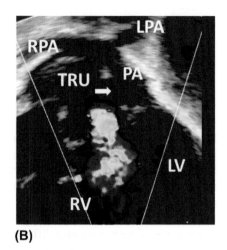

(B)

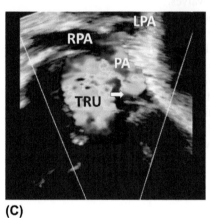

(C)

FIGURE 1

(A) Zoomed apical five-chamber view in a child with type I truncus arteriosus. The pulmonary artery arises from the lateral aspect of the truncus (*arrow*) and then bifurcates. *Asterisk* denotes the outlet ventricular septal defect. (B) Color flow mapping demonstrating severe truncal valve regurgitation. (C) The systolic flow across the truncal valve is mildly turbulent, but this is in the context of a significant truncal regurgitation. *Arrow* indicates flow from the truncus to the pulmonary artery. *LPA*, pulmonary artery; *LV*, left ventricle; *PA*, pulmonary artery; *RA*, right atrium; *RPA*, right pulmonary artery; *RV*, right ventricle; *TRU*, truncus.

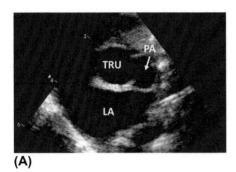
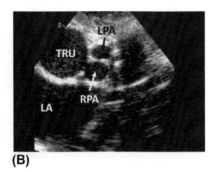

(A)　　　　　　　　　　　(B)

FIGURE 2

Left subclavicular view in a patient with type I truncus arteriosus. (A) Note the origin of the pulmonary artery from the side of the truncus. (B) Subsequent division of the pulmonary artery into its branches. *LA*, left atrium; *LPA*, pulmonary artery; *PA*, pulmonary artery; *RPA*, right pulmonary artery; *TRU*, truncus.

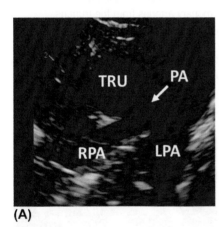
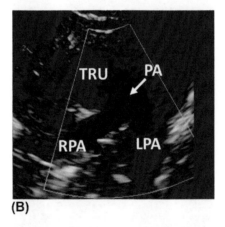

(A)　　　　　　　　　　　(B)

FIGURE 3

(A) Zoomed left subclavicular view in a child with type I truncus arteriosus. Note the presence of a short segment pulmonary artery arising from the truncus and its bifurcation into the right and left pulmonary arteries. (B) Corresponding color flow mapping in the same patient. *LPA*, pulmonary artery; *PA*, pulmonary artery; *RPA*, right pulmonary artery; *TRU*, truncus.

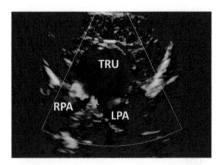

FIGURE 4

Zoomed left subclavicular view in a patient with type II truncus arteriosus. The branch pulmonary arteries have close, but separate origins from the truncus. *LPA*, pulmonary artery; *RPA*, right pulmonary artery; *TRU*, truncus.

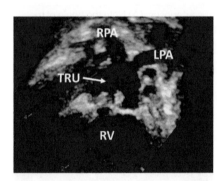

FIGURE 5

Type II truncus arteriosus seen from a zoomed apical five-chamber view. Note the separate origins of the branch pulmonary arteries from the truncus, adjacent to each other. The truncal valve is dysplastic and thickened. *LPA*, pulmonary artery; *LV*, left ventricle; *RPA*, right pulmonary artery; *TRU*, truncus.

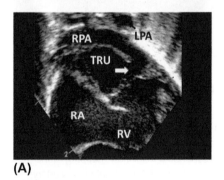
(A)

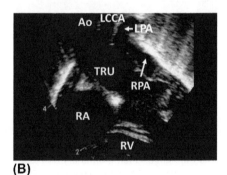
(B)

FIGURE 6

(A) Subcostal five-chamber view illustrating the origin of the right pulmonary artery from the left side of the truncus (*arrow*). The right pulmonary artery then takes a rightward course. (B) The left pulmonary artery originates at a higher level, close to the left common carotid artery, distant from the right pulmonary artery. This child had a right-sided aortic arch with aberrant left subclavian artery (not visualized in this figure). *Ao*, aorta; *LCCA*, left common carotid artery; *LPA*, pulmonary artery; *RA*, right atrium; *RPA*, right pulmonary artery; *RV*, right ventricle; *TRU*, truncus.

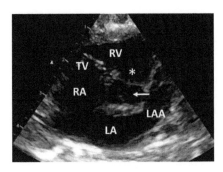

FIGURE 7

Parasternal short-axis view demonstrating a bicommissural (bicuspid) truncal valve (*arrow*) and a large outlet ventricular septal defect (*asterisk*). *LA*, left atrium; *LAA*, left atrial appendage; *RA*, right atrium; *RV*, right ventricle; *TV*, tricuspid valve.

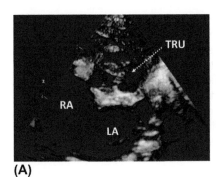

(A)

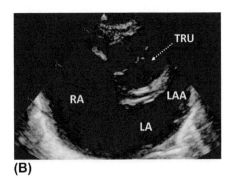

(B)

FIGURE 8

(A) Parasternal short-axis view illustrating a severely dysplastic tricommissural (tricuspid) truncal valve. Note the thickening of the cusps. (B) Quadricommissural (quadricuspid) truncal valve seen in a different patient. *LA*, left atrium; *LAA*, left atrial appendage; *RA*, right atrium; *TRU*, truncal valve.

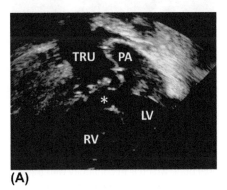

(A)

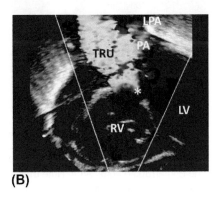

(B)

FIGURE 9

(A) Zoomed modified subcostal short-axis view in a newborn with type I truncus arteriosus (pulmonary artery origin from truncus not shown) and severe dysplasia and thickening of the truncal valve. The *asterisk* indicates an outlet ventricular septal defect. The truncal valve is overriding the interventricular septum. (B) Color flow mapping illustrating turbulent flow across the valve due to stenosis. *LPA*, pulmonary artery; *LV*, left ventricle; *PA*, pulmonary artery; *RV*, right ventricle; *TRU*, truncus.

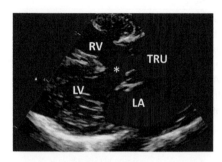

FIGURE 10

Parasternal long-axis view illustrating an outlet ventricular septal defect (*asterisk*) and truncal overriding. In this figure, the truncus is connected predominantly to the right ventricle. *LA*, left atrium; *LV*, left ventricle; *RV*, right ventricle; *TRU*, truncus.

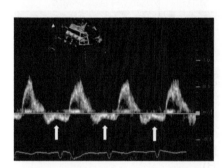

FIGURE 11

Pulsed-wave Doppler of the abdominal aorta from the subcostal view. *Arrows* indicate holodiastolic flow reversal in the aorta, which is driven by low pulmonary vascular resistance. This finding is typically present, among others, in patients with persistent truncus arteriosus.

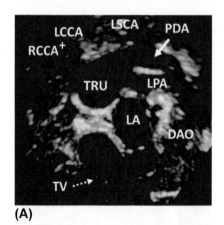

(A)

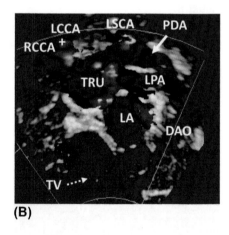

(B)

FIGURE 12

(A) Modified subcostal short-axis view in a newborn with type II truncus arteriosus and type B interrupted aortic arch. Note the large arterial duct, which is in continuity with the descending aorta, forming a (left-sided) ductal arch. The left pulmonary artery arises directly from the truncus. The right and left common carotid arteries have a common origin from the truncus. The left subclavian artery originates from the proximal descending aorta. The child had aberrant right subclavian artery (not shown). (B) Corresponding color flow mapping. *DAo*, descending aorta; *LA*, left atrium; *LCCA*, left common carotid artery; *LPA*, pulmonary artery; *LSCA*, left subclavian artery; *RCCA*, right common carotid artery; *TRU*, truncus; *TV*, tricuspid valve.

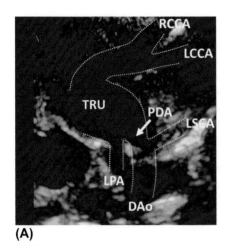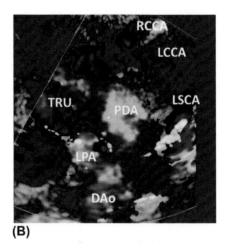

(A) **(B)**

FIGURE 13

(A) The same patient as in Figure 12 with type II truncus arteriosus and type B interrupted aortic arch seen from the suprasternal notch view. The left pulmonary artery originates directly from the truncus. The ascending aorta arises from the truncus and gives rise to the right and left common carotid arteries. The left subclavian artery comes off the ductal arch and is not in continuity with the ascending aorta. The aberrant right subclavian artery is not shown in this figure. (B) Corresponding color flow mapping. *DAo*, descending aorta; *LCCA*, left common carotid artery; *LPA*, pulmonary artery; *LSCA*, left subclavian artery; *PDA*, patent ductus arteriosus; *RCCA*, right common carotid artery; *TRU*, truncus.

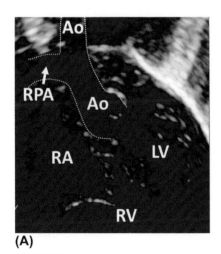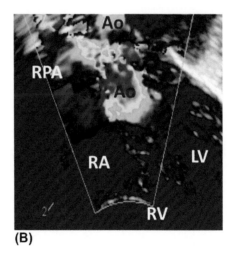

(A) **(B)**

FIGURE 14

(A) Subcostal long-axis view demonstrating the isolated origin of the right pulmonary artery from the ascending aorta (hemitruncus). The origin of the left pulmonary artery from the pulmonary artery is not shown in this figure. (B) Color flow mapping illustrating direct communication between the ascending aorta and the right pulmonary artery. *Ao*, aorta; *LV*, left ventricle; *RA*, right atrium; *RPA*, right pulmonary artery; *RV*, right ventricle.

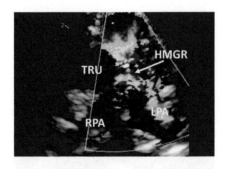

FIGURE 15

Zoomed parasternal short-axis view showing a stenotic homograft several years after surgical repair of truncus arteriosus. The homograft was used to connect the right ventricle to the pulmonary vasculature. Chronic degenerative changes, which usually occur over a number of years, result in homograft obstruction and/or regurgitation and lead to the necessity of its replacement. *HMGR*, homograft; *LPA*, pulmonary artery; *RPA*, right pulmonary artery; *TRU*, truncus; *LPA*, pulmonary artery; *RPA*, right pulmonary artery; *TRU*, truncus.

Functionally single ventricle

15

Functionally single ventricle is an umbrella term for a group of severe congenital heart defects that are not suitable for the creation of a biventricular circulation and that can only be palliated using a univentricular approach. This is mainly due to the hypoplasia of one of the ventricles and the inability to generate adequate cardiac output, as in **hypoplastic left heart syndrome, pulmonary atresia with intact ventricular septum,** or **unbalanced defect of the atrio-ventricular septum.** In other cases, there is a univentricular atrio-ventricular connection, as in atrio-ventricular valve atresia (**mitral** or **tricuspid atresia**) or in **double inlet ventricle.** Finally, some patients with large or multiple ventricular septal defects may also require univentricular palliation.

These defects are becoming increasingly rare because of the progress in prenatal screening and account for approximately 5% of the congenital heart defects. Surgical palliation in patients with functionally single ventricle is a multistep process aiming to create a total cavo-pulmonary connection (Fontan circulation). The univentricular pathway is burdened with significant morbidity and mortality due to the number of differences from normal biventricular circulation.

Hypoplastic left heart syndrome

Hypoplastic left heart (HLH) syndrome is a common term for a group of cardiac defects characterized by underdevelopment of the left-sided heart structures. In extreme cases, there is mitral and aortic atresia and the left ventricular cavity is not detectable. At the other end of the spectrum, the mitral and aortic valves are stenotic, and the left ventricle has borderline dimensions, but is unable to sustain the systemic circulation.

It is important to mention that a small but functionally adequate left ventricle may be present in other malformations such as coarctation of the aorta (see Chapter 17, Figure 10). The presence of ventricular imbalance is usually the result of altered fetal hemodynamics caused by changes in preload or afterload and does not determine the intrinsic ventricular hypoplasia. In some patients with a borderline left ventricle, the decision between univentricular or biventricular repair is particularly challenging.

In hypoplastic left heart syndrome, the left ventricle is typically very dysfunctional. Another hallmark of the disease is the presence of endocardial fibroelastosis, which affects the growth and the function of the left ventricle. The aortic arch is always hypoplastic and coarctation of the aorta is often present. There is the retrograde filling of the ascending aorta from the duct due to negligible or no blood flow across the aortic valve and the circulation is thus duct dependant.

Atlas of Pediatric Echocardiography. https://doi.org/10.1016/B978-0-323-75981-6.00020-0

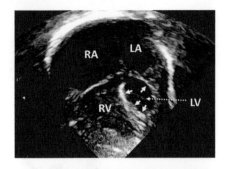

FIGURE 1

Apical four-chamber view in a neonate with hypoplastic left heart syndrome and severe mitral and aortic stenosis. The left ventricle is diminutive, nonapex forming, and dysfunctional. Note the presence of endocardial fibroelastosis (*arrows*). *LA*, left atrium; *LV*, left ventricle; *RA*, right atrium; *RV*, right ventricle.

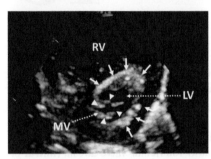

FIGURE 2

Parasternal short-axis view in a patient with hypoplastic left heart syndrome demonstrating a severely reduced mitral valve orifice area (*arrowheads*) and endocardial fibroelastosis (*arrows*). *LV*, left ventricle; *MV*, mitral valve; *RV*, right ventricle.

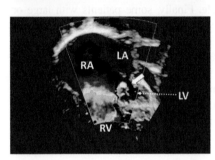

FIGURE 3

Apical four-chamber view in a child with severe hypoplasia of the left ventricle. There is detectable flow across the very stenotic mitral valve (*arrow*) on color flow mapping. Note the right atrial and ventricular dilatation. *LA*, left atrium; *LV*, left ventricle; *RA*, right atrium; *RV*, right ventricle.

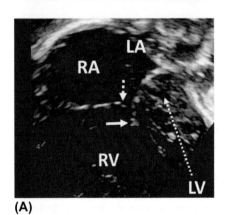

(A)

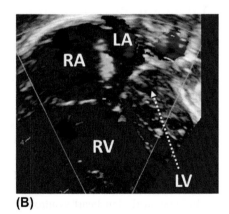

(B)

FIGURE 4

(A) Apical four-chamber view in a newborn with hypoplastic left heart syndrome and a very diminutive left ventricle. Note the incomplete coaptation between the anterior and septal leaflets of the tricuspid valve caused by the reduced motion of the fixed septal leaflet. *Dotted arrow* indicates the tip of the antero-superior tricuspid valve leaflet, *plain arrow* the tip of the septal tricuspid valve leaflet. (B) As a consequence, there is severe tricuspid regurgitation contributing to the dilatation of the right-sided chambers. *LA*, left atrium; *LV*, left ventricle; *RA*, right atrium; *RV*, right ventricle.

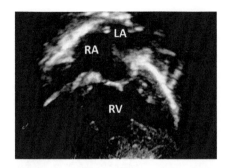

FIGURE 5

Apical four-chamber view in a neonate with hypoplastic left heart syndrome and mitral and aortic atresia. The mitral valve is absent and no left ventricular cavity is visible. The right atrium and ventricle are dilated. *LA*, left atrium; *RA*, right atrium; *RV*, right ventricle.

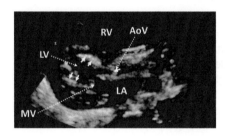

FIGURE 6

Parasternal long-axis view demonstrating hypoplasia of the left ventricle. The aortic and mitral valves are small and severely stenotic. There is hyperechogenicity of the endocardium consistent with endocardial fibroelastosis (*arrows*). *AoV*, aortic valve; *LA*, left atrium; *LV*, left ventricle; *MV*, mitral valve; *RV*, right ventricle.

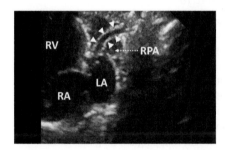

FIGURE 7

Modified suprasternal notch view in a neonate with hypoplastic left heart syndrome and mitral and aortic atresia. *Arrowheads* indicate the very hypoplastic ascending aorta, the size of which is much smaller than the diameter of the right pulmonary artery. *LA*, left atrium; *RA*, right atrium; *RPA*, right pulmonary artery; *RV*, right ventricle.

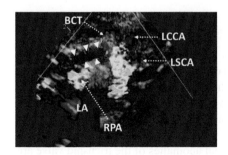

FIGURE 8

Suprasternal notch view in a patient with hypoplastic left heart syndrome and aortic atresia showing a severely hypoplastic ascending aorta (*arrowheads*). Color flow mapping demonstrating retrograde filling of the aortic arch from the duct. *BCT*, brachiocephalic trunk; *LA*, left atrium; *LCCA*, left common carotid artery; *LSCA*, left subclavian artery; *RPA*, right pulmonary artery.

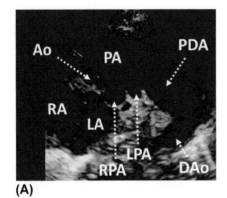 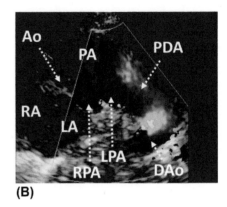

(A) **(B)**

FIGURE 9

(A) High parasternal short-axis view in a newborn with hypoplastic left heart syndrome. Note the severe hypoplasia of the ascending aorta. Due to an infusion of prostaglandins, the arterial duct, which is continuous with the descending aorta, is very large. (B) Corresponding color flow mapping showing a right-to-left shunt across the duct. Retrograde filling of the aortic arch from the duct is not shown in this figure. *Ao*, aorta; *DAo*, descending aorta; *LA*, left atrium; *LPA*, left pulmonary artery; *PA*, pulmonary artery; *PDA*, patent ductus arteriosus; *RA*, right atrium; *RPA*, right pulmonary artery.

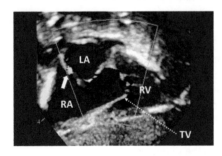

FIGURE 10

Patients with hypoplastic left heart syndrome are usually born with a restrictive interatrial communication, as illustrated in this figure. It is thought that intrauterine restriction at the atrial level decreases blood flow to the left side of the heart, thus contributes to its underdevelopment. Subcostal view with color flow mapping showing restrictive left-to-right shunt across a small patent foramen ovale (*arrow*). *LA*, left atrium; *RA*, right atrium; *RV*, right ventricle; *TV*, tricuspid valve.

Pulmonary atresia with intact ventricular septum

In pulmonary atresia with intact ventricular septum, the atresia of the right ventricular outflow tract is either due to the fusion of the pulmonary valve cusps (membranous atresia) or to muscular obliteration of the infundibulum (muscular atresia). The size of the right ventricle varies from severe hypoplasia to a reasonably well-developed chamber. The absence of the trabecular or outlet portions of the right ventricle is associated with worse outcome.

In this condition, anatomical and functional anomalies of the tricuspid valve are common and include various degrees of hypoplasia, stenosis or regurgitation.

Another feature of the disease it the development of coronary sinusoids, especially in the absence of tricuspid regurgitation. Coronary sinusoids allow decompression of the right ventricle, but in some cases lead to the progressive development of coronary stenoses and occlusions. This results in the dependence of the right ventricle for coronary perfusion, which is associated with poor prognosis.

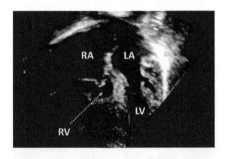

FIGURE 11

Apical four-chamber view demonstrating severe hypoplasia and hypertrophy of the right ventricle in a child with pulmonary atresia with intact ventricular septum. The tricuspid valve is dysplastic and barely opens in diastole. Note the complete opening of the mitral valve. *LA*, left atrium; *LV*, left ventricle; *RA*, right atrium; *RV*, right ventricle.

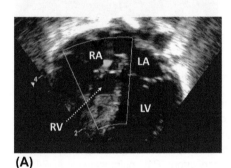

(A)

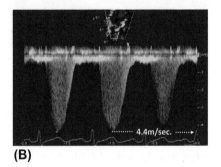

(B)

FIGURE 12

(A) Apical four-chamber view in a child with pulmonary atresia with intact ventricular septum. Color flow mapping demonstrating moderate tricuspid regurgitation decompressing the diminutive right ventricle. Note the absence of coronary sinusoids. (B) Continuous-wave Doppler of the tricuspid valve showing the regurgitant signal only. The tricuspid regurgitation peak velocity is high (4.4 m/s), consistent with systemic level (systolic) right ventricular pressure. *LA*, left atrium; *LV*, left ventricle; *RA*, right atrium; *RV*, right ventricle.

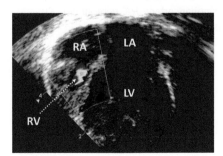

FIGURE 13

Apical four-chamber view with color flow mapping illustrating tricuspid inflow in a child with pulmonary atresia with intact ventricular septum. Note the hypoplasia of the right ventricle and tricuspid valve. *LA*, left atrium; *LV*, left ventricle; *RA*, right atrium; *RV*, right ventricle.

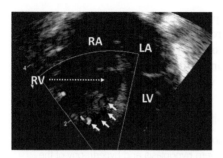

FIGURE 14

Patient with pulmonary atresia with intact ventricular septum. Apical four-chamber view with color flow mapping demonstrating coronary sinusoids in the right ventricular myocardium (*arrows*). *LA*, left atrium; *LV*, left ventricle; *RA*, right atrium; *RV*, right ventricle.

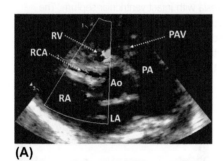

(A)

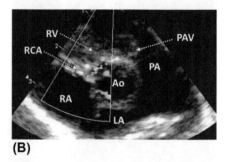

(B)

FIGURE 15

Parasternal short axis view in a child with pulmonary atresia with intact ventricular septum. There is bidirectional flow in the right coronary artery, which suggests the coronary circulation is dependent upon the right ventricle. (A) Color flow mapping demonstrating antegrade flow in the right coronary artery. (B) Retrograde right coronary artery flow. *Ao*, aorta; *LA*, left atrium; *PA*, pulmonary artery; *PAV*, pulmonary valve; *RA*, right atrium; *RCA*, right coronary artery; *RV*, right ventricle.

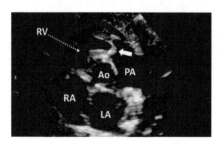

FIGURE 16

Parasternal short-axis view in a child with membranous atresia of the pulmonary valve (*arrow*) and intact ventricular septum. *Ao*, aorta; *LA*, left atrium; *PA*, pulmonary artery; *RA*, right atrium; *RV*, right ventricle.

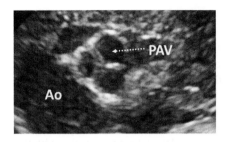

FIGURE 17

Zoomed suprasternal notch view demonstrating a well developed but atretic pulmonary valve. The valve is tricuspid and there is a complete fusion of the cusps. *Ao*, aorta; *PAV*, pulmonary valve.

Unbalanced atrio-ventricular septal defect

Unbalanced atrio-ventricular septal defects account for approximately 10% of all atrio-ventricular septal defects. The hallmark of the disease is hypoplasia of one of the ventricles and usually the outflow tract as well. There is malalignment of the atrio-ventricular junction that defines the dominant chamber. Abnormalities of the ventriculo-arterial junction are often present in this condition.

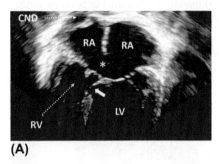

(A)

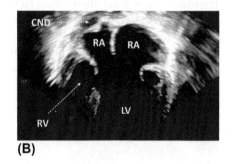

(B)

FIGURE 18

(A) Apical four-chamber view demonstrating an unbalanced atrio-ventricular (AV) septal defect in a child with right atrial isomerism. The atrial and ventricular septae are malaligned, with the ventricular septum displaced to the right. There is a dominant left and hypoplastic right ventricle. The *asterisk* denotes an ostium primum atrial septal defect, the *arrow* indicates a ventricular septal defect. Note the presence of an extracardiac conduit due to the previous completion of a total cavo-pulmonary connection. (B) Diastolic opening of the common AV valve in the same patient. *CND*, extracardiac conduit; *LV*, left ventricle; *RA*, right atrium; *RV*, right ventricle.

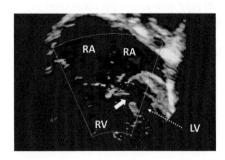

FIGURE 19

An unbalanced atrio-ventricular (AV) septal defect in a patient with right atrial isomerism and hypoplasia of the left ventricle. Note the left AV valve regurgitation, the jet is directed into the left-sided right atrium. *Arrow* indicates an inlet ventricular septal defect. *LV*, left ventricle; *RA*, right atrium; *RV*, right ventricle.

Tricuspid atresia

Tricuspid atresia is a rare cardiac defect characterized either by the presence of an imperforate valve, or far more often, by the absence of the right atrio-ventricular connection. In the latter case, the floor of the right atrium and the right ventricle are completely disconnected by the interventricular sulcus. There is an obligatory right-to-left shunt at atrial level and enlargement of the left-sided chambers taking both the systemic and pulmonary venous return.

The right ventricle is usually diminutive, has no inlet, and communicates with the left ventricle through a ventricular septal defect. The ventriculo-arterial connection is most commonly concordant and less often discordant. In some cases, there is valvar pulmonary stenosis or atresia. A restrictive interventricular communication can cause obstruction at subvalvar level and is typically associated with coarctation of the aorta in patients with discordant great arteries (aorta arising from the right ventricle).

From a clinical point of view, patients with tricuspid atresia can be divided into three different categories. Neonates with **tricuspid atresia and severe right ventricular outflow tract obstruction (RVOTO)** usually have a duct dependant circulation. Those with **mild-to-moderate RVOTO** may remain hemodynamically stable, sometimes even for several years. Patients with an **unobstructed right ventricular outflow tract and a large ventricular septal defect** usually develop clinical signs of high pulmonary blood flow in the first few weeks of life.

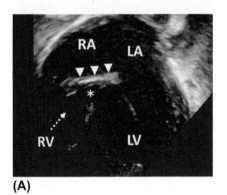 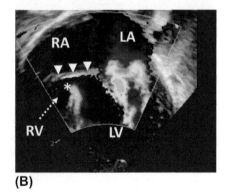

(A)   **(B)**

FIGURE 20

(A) Apical four-chamber view in a child with absent right atrio-ventricular connection (*arrowheads*). The *asterisk* indicates the ventricular septal defect connecting the systemic left ventricle with the rudimentary right ventricle. (B) Color flow mapping demonstrating flow across the mitral valve and the ventricular septal defect. *LA*, left atrium; *LV*, left ventricle; *RA*, right atrium; *RV*, right ventricle.

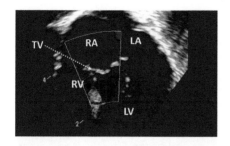

FIGURE 21

Imperforate tricuspid valve seen from the apical four-chamber view. Unlike the mitral valve, the tricuspid valve does not open in diastole. There is no detectable flow across the atretic valve on color flow mapping. The *asterisk* corresponds to a ventricular septal defect. *LA*, left atrium; *LV*, left ventricle; *RA*, right atrium; *RV*, right ventricle; *TV*, tricuspid valve.

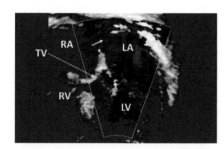

FIGURE 22

Zoomed apical four-chamber view with color flow mapping demonstrating a right-to-left shunt at atrial level (*arrow*) due to the presence of an imperforate tricuspid valve. *LA*, left atrium; *LV*, left ventricle; *RA*, right atrium; *RV*, right ventricle; *TV*, tricuspid valve.

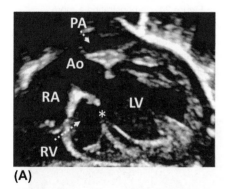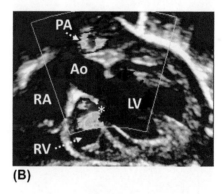

(A) (B)

FIGURE 23

(A) Tricuspid atresia with concordant ventriculo-arterial connection visualized from the subcostal long-axis view. The rudimentary right ventricle communicates with the systemic left ventricle through a ventricular septal defect (*asterisk*). (B) Obligatory left-to-right shunt across the defect on color flow mapping. *Ao*, aorta; *LV*, left ventricle; *PA*, pulmonary artery; *RA*, right atrium; *RV*, right ventricle.

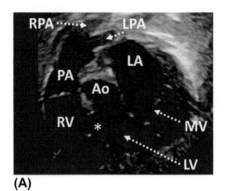
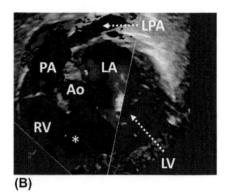

(A)   **(B)**

FIGURE 24

(A) Subcostal short-axis view showing concordant ventriculo-arterial connection in a patient with tricuspid atresia. The pulmonary artery is more anterior compared to the aorta and arises from the rudimentary right ventricle. Both ventricles are connected through a large ventricular septal defect (*asterisk*). The pulmonary valve is not stenotic. (B) Color flow mapping illustrating a left-to-right shunt across the unrestrictive ventricular communication. *Ao*, aorta; *LA*, left atrium; *LPA*, left pulmonary artery; *LV*, left ventricle; *MV*, mitral valve; *PA*, pulmonary artery; *RPA*, right pulmonary artery; *RV*, right ventricle.

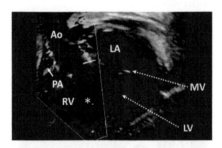

FIGURE 25

Subcostal short-axis view in the same child as in Figure 24, demonstrating a more posterior origin of the aorta compared to the pulmonary artery. *Ao*, aorta; *LA*, left atrium; *LV*, left ventricle; *MV*, mitral valve; *PA*, pulmonary artery; *RV*, right ventricle.

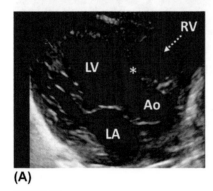
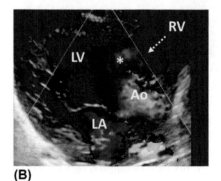

(A)   **(B)**

FIGURE 26

(A) Parasternal long-axis view in a child with tricuspid atresia and concordant ventriculo-arterial connection. The right ventricle is diminutive and anterior to the left ventricle. *Asterisk* indicates the ventricular septal defect. (B) Color flow mapping illustrating the left-to-right shunt across the ventricular septal defect (*asterisk*). *Ao*, aorta; *LA*, left atrium; *LV*, left ventricle; *RV*, right ventricle.

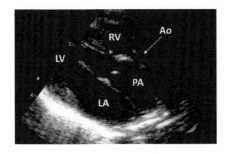

FIGURE 27

Parasternal long-axis view in a patient with tricuspid atresia and ventriculo-arterial discordance. Note the "double barrel shotgun" appearance of the great arteries. The ventricular septal defect (*asterisk*) is restrictive, causing a significant subaortic obstruction. As a result, the aorta is hypoplastic. In addition, there was coarctation of the aorta (not shown).

Ao, aorta; *LA*, left atrium; *LV*, left ventricle; *PA*, pulmonary artery; *RV*, right ventricle.

Double inlet ventricle

The term **double inlet ventricle** refers to a cardiac malformation in which both atria are connected to one dominant ventricle via one common or two separate atrio-ventricular valves. These hearts usually have a second, rudimentary chamber that has no inlet and communicates with the dominant ventricle through a ventricular septal defect.

In **double inlet left ventricle (DILV)**, the dominant ventricle has anatomical features of the left ventricle and the rudimentary chamber is anterior. If the dominant ventricular chamber is the right ventricle, the term **double inlet right ventricle (DIRV)** is used. The latter is characterized by an inferior rudimentary chamber. In some patients, the morphology of the dominant ventricle cannot be determined and the rudimentary chamber may be absent.

Typically, one great artery, which may be stenotic or atretic, arises from both the dominant and rudimentary chamber. The great arteries are either normally related, or there is right or left anterior position of the aorta. The most common type of double inlet ventricle is DILV with left anterior aorta, followed by DILV with right anterior aorta. DIRV is a rare cardiac defect.

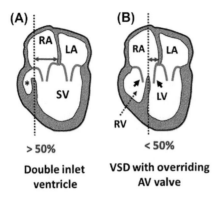

(A) >50%
Double inlet ventricle

(B) <50%
VSD with overriding AV valve

FIGURE 28

Difference between double inlet ventricle with two separate atrio-ventricular (AV) valves and ventricular septal defect (VSD) with overriding AV valve. (A) Double inlet ventricle is defined by >50% commitment of both AV valves to one dominant ventricular chamber. *Asterisk* indicates the rudimentary chamber. (B) If there is <50% commitment of one of the AV valves to the contralateral ventricle, the term ventricular septal defect (VSD) with overriding AV valve

is used. The latter is typically associated with AV valve straddling, that is, attachment of the valve to both sides of the interventricular septum (*arrows*).

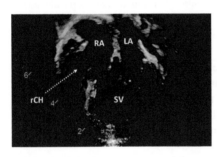

FIGURE 29

Double inlet left ventricle seen from the apical four-chamber view. Both atrio-ventricular valves are committed to a single ventricular chamber that has left ventricular morphology. Note the presence of a rudimentary chamber that communicates with the dominant ventricle through a ventricular septal

defect. *LV*, left ventricle; *RA*, right atrium; *rCh*, rudimentary chamber; *SV*, dominant ventricle.

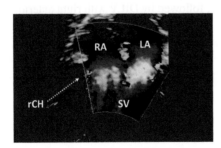

FIGURE 30

Apical four-chamber view with color flow mapping showing blood flow across both atrio-ventricular valves into the dominant ventricular chamber. Note the right-sided rudimentary chamber. *LA*, left atrium; *RA*, right atrium; *rCh*, rudimentary chamber; *SV*, dominant ventricle.

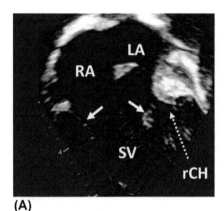 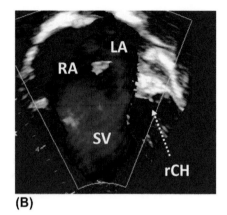

(A)   **(B)**

FIGURE 31

(A) Double inlet ventricle with common atrio-ventricular valve seen from the apical four-chamber view. Note the presence of a common atrio-ventricular valve (*arrows*) connecting both atria with one dominant ventricular chamber. The rudimentary chamber is to the left of the dominant ventricle. (B) Color flow mapping illustrating blood flow across the common atrio-ventricular valve into the dominant ventricle. *LA*, left atrium; *RA*, right atrium; *rCh*, rudimentary chamber; *SV*, dominant ventricle.

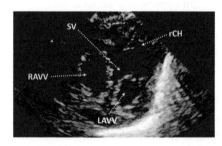

FIGURE 32

Patient with double inlet left ventricle and left anterior position of the rudimentary chamber. Parasternal short-axis view demonstrating commitment of both atrio-ventricular valves to the dominant ventricle. *LAVV*, left atrio-ventricular valve; *RAVV*, right atrio-ventricular valve; *rCh*, rudimentary chamber; *SV*, dominant ventricle.

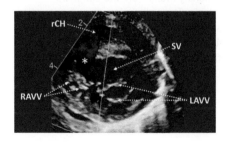

FIGURE 33

Parasternal short-axis view in a child with double inlet left ventricle and ventriculo-arterial concordance (not shown). Color flow mapping demonstrating blood flow across the ventricular septal defect (*asterisk*). The direction of the shunt is from the dominant ventricle to the right anterior rudimentary chamber. *LAVV*, left atrio-ventricular valve; *RAVV*, right atrio-ventricular valve; *rCh*, rudimentary chamber; *SV*, dominant ventricle.

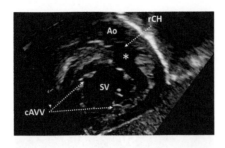

FIGURE 34

Double inlet ventricle with common atrio-ventricular valve seen from the subcostal short-axis view. The common atrio-ventricular valve opens into the dominant ventricular chamber. The *asterisk* indicates a ventricular septal defect connecting the dominant ventricular chamber to the left-sided rudimentary (subaortic) chamber. The ventriculo-arterial connection was discordant in this child. *Ao*, aorta; *cAVV*, common atrio-ventricular valve; *rCh*, rudimentary chamber; *SV*, dominant ventricle.

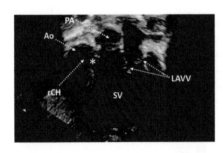

FIGURE 35

Apical five-chamber view demonstrating the origin of the aorta and the pulmonary artery in a child with double inlet left ventricle. The ventriculo-arterial connection is discordant, with the pulmonary artery arising from the dominant ventricle and the aorta from the right-sided rudimentary outlet chamber. *Asterisk* indicates the ventricular septal defect. *LAVV*, left atrio-ventricular valve; *rCH*, rudimentary chamber; *SV*, dominant ventricle.

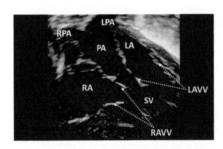

FIGURE 36

Double inlet left ventricle with ventriculo-arterial discordance. Subcostal five-chamber view showing the origin of the pulmonary artery from the dominant ventricle. The rudimentary chamber is not visualized in this figure. *LA*, left atrium; *LAVV*, left atrio-ventricular valve; *LPA*, left pulmonary artery; *PA*, pulmonary artery; *RA*, right atrium; *RAVV*, right atrio-ventricular valve; *RPA*, right pulmonary artery; *SV*, dominant ventricle.

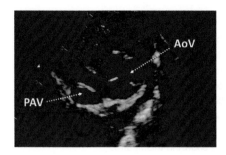

FIGURE 37

Zoomed modified suprasternal notch view in a child with double inlet left ventricle, ventriculo-arterial discordance, and valvar pulmonary stenosis. The pulmonary valve (PAV) is small and bicommissural (bicuspid). The aortic valve (AoV) is anterior and to the left of the pulmonary valve.

Interventions for functionally single ventricle patients

If eligible, patients with functionally single ventricle undergo staged surgical palliation, which usually involves three steps. The first stage of palliation consists of a heterogenous group of interventions. The creation of a shunt (modified Blalock-Taussig shunt, Sano shunt, etc.) is required in patients with insufficient pulmonary blood supply. On the other hand, pulmonary artery banding is performed in children with excessive pulmonary blood flow, as low pulmonary vascular resistance is essential in single ventricle physiology. The creation of a connection of the pulmonary artery to the ascending aorta (Damus—Kaye—Stansel procedure) is indicated in children with obstruction to the systemic outflow.

The second stage of palliation, which is usually carried out around the age of 3—6 months, consists in the creation of an anastomosis between the superior vena cava and the right pulmonary artery (Glenn procedure or bidirectional cavo-pulmonary anastomosis). The last stage involves connection of the inferior vena cava to the right pulmonary artery, usually via an extracardiac conduit, thereby creating a total cavo-pulmonary connection (TCPC). This generally happens at around 3 years old.

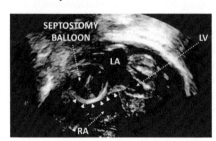

FIGURE 38

Subcostal four-chamber view in a patient with hypoplastic left heart syndrome and restrictive atrial communication undergoing balloon atrial septostomy. Note the presence of the septostomy balloon in the left atrium pulling the atrial septum (*arrowheads*) into the right atrium. *LA*, left atrium; *LV*, left ventricle; *RA*, right atrium.

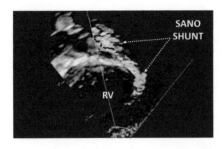

FIGURE 39

Child with hypoplastic left heart syndrome after first stage palliation (Norwood procedure). Zoomed subcostal view with color flow mapping demonstrating a Sano shunt. The Sano shunt is a Gore-Tex conduit connecting the systemic right ventricle (RV) to the distal stump of the pulmonary artery (not shown in this figure).

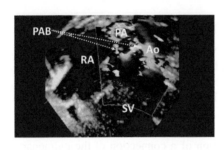

FIGURE 40

Patient with double inlet left ventricle, discordant ventriculo-arterial connection and anterior aorta arising from the hypoplastic (left-sided) rudimentary chamber. Note the presence of a pulmonary artery band restricting the blood flow across the pulmonary artery. Color flow mapping demonstrating flow turbulence starting at the level of the band. *Ao*, aorta; *PA*, pulmonary artery; *PAB*, pulmonary artery band; *RA*, right atrium; *SV*, dominant ventricle.

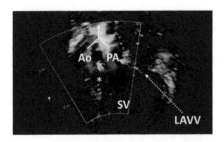

FIGURE 41

Zoomed apical five-chamber view in a child with double inlet left ventricle and ventriculo-arterial discordance. Color flow mapping demonstrating an anastomosis (*Y shaped arrow*) between the proximal pulmonary artery and the aorta (Damus—Kaye—Stansel or DKS procedure). This intervention is performed in patients with obstruction to the systemic outflow, which is usually caused, as in this case, by a restrictive subaortic ventricular septal defect (*asterisk*). *Ao*, aorta; *LAVV*, left atrioventricular valve; *PA*, pulmonary artery; *SV*, dominant ventricle.

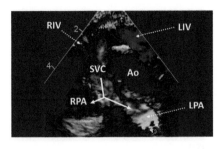

FIGURE 42

Glenn shunt (also known as bidirectional cavo-pulmonary anastomosis) seen from the suprasternal notch view (frontal plane). Note the end-to-side anastomosis between the superior vena cava and the right pulmonary artery (*Y shaped arrow*). *Ao*, aorta; *LIV*, left innominate vein; *LPA*, left pulmonary artery; *RIV*, right innominate vein; *RPA*, right pulmonary artery; *SVC*, superior vena cava.

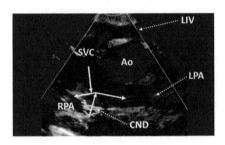

FIGURE 43

Total cavo-pulmonary connection (Fontan procedure) seen from the suprasternal notch view (frontal plane). Color flow mapping demonstrating the anastomosis between both the superior and inferior venae cavae and the right pulmonary artery (*arrows*). The inferior vena cava is connected to the right pulmonary artery via an extracardiac conduit. LIV left innominate vein; *CND*, extracardiac conduit; *LPA*, left pulmonary artery; *RPA*, right pulmonary artery; *SVC*, superior vena cava.

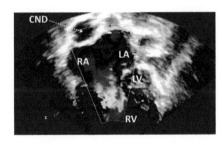

FIGURE 44

Patient with hypoplastic left heart syndrome after completion of the total cavo-pulmonary connection. Apical four-chamber view showing a nonfenestrated extracardiac conduit located behind the right atrium. Note the absence of interatrial septum due to previous surgical septectomy. *CND*, extracardiac conduit; *LA*, left atrium; *LV*, left ventricle; *RA*, right atrium; *RV*, right ventricle.

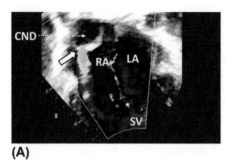
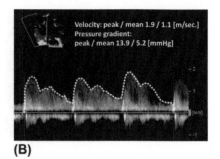

(A) **(B)**

FIGURE 45

In some patients, a small fenestration is created between the extracardiac conduit and the right atrium at the time of completion of the total cavo-pulmonary connection (TCPC). This helps to decrease the venous pressure in the TCPC system. (A) Fenestrated TCPC in a child with double inlet left ventricle seen from a zoomed apical four-chamber view. The *arrow* indicates a fenestration with blood flow from the conduit to the right atrium. (B) The mean pressure gradient across the fenestration reflects the transpulmonary gradient and can be measured by continuous-wave Doppler (5.2 mmHg in this example). *CND*, extracardiac conduit; *LA*, left atrium; *RA*, right atrium; *SV*, dominant ventricle.

Patent ductus arteriosus (PDA) and aorto-pulmonary window

16

Patent ductus arteriosus (PDA)

In utero, the ductus arteriosus diverts part of the pulmonary blood flow to the descending aorta. This leads to an increase in placental perfusion at the expense of nonfunctioning lungs. In most children, the ductus arteriosus closes spontaneously soon after birth, but in some cases, especially in preterm infants, it may remain open. On the other hand, in patients with critical cardiac malformations and duct dependant circulation, an infusion of prostaglandins is necessary to maintain its patency.

The persistence of a large patent ductus arteriosus (PDA) in the context of low pulmonary vascular resistance will result in left heart volume overload, pulmonary overcirculation, and progressive development of pulmonary hypertension. The direction of shunt and the velocity of blood flow across the ductus will reflect the difference between the pulmonary and aortic pressures. Treatment of a PDA consists in transcatheter closure or surgical ligation and is indicated in symptomatic children, especially in preterm infants, who have failed medical therapy.

Atlas of Pediatric Echocardiography. https://doi.org/10.1016/B978-0-323-75981-6.00009-1

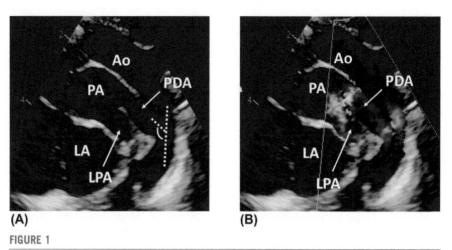

FIGURE 1

(A) Suprasternal notch view demonstrating of the entire course of the PDA. Due to the fact that in utero the blood is shunted from the pulmonary artery to the aorta, the PDA inserts into the aorta at an obtuse angle (*dotted lines*). (B) Color flow mapping showing a left-to-right shunt across the PDA. *Ao*, aorta; *LA*, left atrium; *PA*, pulmonary artery.

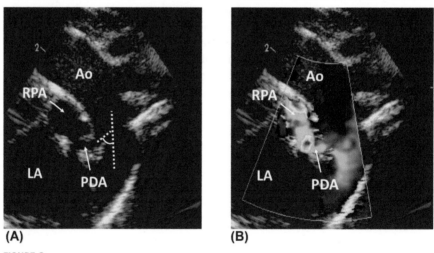

FIGURE 2

(A) Suprasternal notch view in a newborn with severe pulmonary stenosis. In contrast to Figure 1, the PDA arises from the aorta at an acute angle (*dotted lines*). In patients with significantly reduced or no antegrade flow across the pulmonary valve in utero, the developing lungs are supplied retrogradely from the aorta. This results in a reverse orientation of the duct. (B) Color flow mapping demonstrating a left-to-right shunt across the PDA. *Ao*, aorta; *LA*, left atrium; *RPA*, right pulmonary artery.

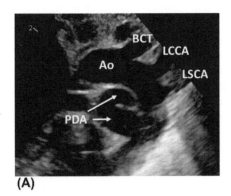
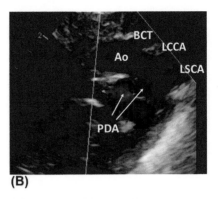

(A)   **(B)**

FIGURE 3

(A) Suprasternal notch view illustrating serpentine course of the PDA in a newborn with critical pulmonary stenosis. The PDA joins the pulmonary artery after a series of turns (the pulmonary end of the PDA is not shown). Tortuous PDAs are often seen in patients with right-sided obstructive lesions. (B) Color flow mapping in the same patient. *Ao*, aorta; *BCT*, brachiocephalic trunk; *LCCA*, left common carotid artery; *LCCA*, left subclavian artery.

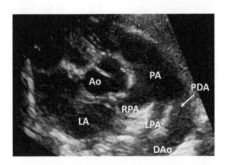

FIGURE 4

Entire course of the PDA shown from the parasternal short-axis view. *Ao*, aorta; *DAo*, descending aorta; *LA*, left atrium; *LPA*, left pulmonary artery; *PA*, pulmonary artery; *RPA*, right pulmonary artery.

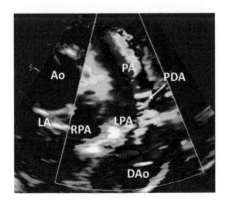

FIGURE 5

Left-to-right shunt across the PDA visualized on color flow mapping from a zoomed parasternal short-axis view. *Ao*, aorta; *DAo*, decending aorta; *LA*, left atrium; *LPA*, left pulmonary artery; *PA*, pulmonary artery; *RPA*, right pulmonary artery.

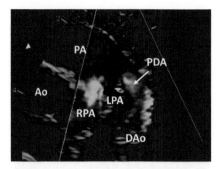

FIGURE 6

Parasternal short-axis view in a neonate with persistent pulmonary hypertension of the newborn (PPHN). Color flow mapping demonstrating a right-to-left shunt across the PDA. *Ao,* aorta; *DAo,* decending aorta; *LA,* left atrium; *LPA,* left pulmonary artery; *PA,* pulmonary artery; *RPA,* right pulmonary artery.

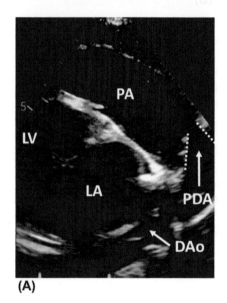

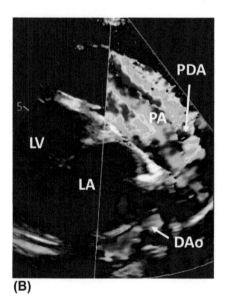

(A) (B)

FIGURE 7

(A) Modified parasternal short-axis view. PDA has a typical conical shape (*dotted lines*), with the aortic end being broader than the pulmonary end. (B) Color flow mapping showing restricted blood flow across the PDA starting at the level of the pulmonary end, which represents the narrowest part. *DAo,* descending aorta; *LA,* left atrium; *PA,* pulmonary artery; *PDA,* arterial duct.

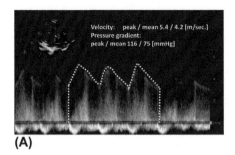

Velocity: peak / mean 5.4 / 4.2 [m/sec.]
Pressure gradient:
peak / mean 116 / 75 [mmHg]

(A)

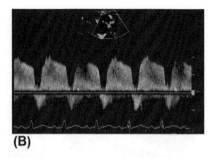

(B)

FIGURE 8

Continuous-wave Doppler of the PDA from the parasternal short-axis view. (A) High-velocity left-to-right shunt consistent with low pulmonary artery pressure. In this example, the peak pressure gradient between the aorta and the pulmonary artery is 116 mmHg. (B) Low-velocity bidirectional shunt (brief systolic right-to-left) in a neonate with persistent pulmonary hypertension of the newborn (PPHN) and systemic level pulmonary artery pressure.

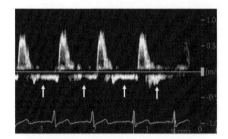

FIGURE 9

Pulsed-wave Doppler of the abdominal aorta from the subcostal view in a child with a hemodynamically significant PDA. The *arrows* indicate holodiastolic flow reversal driven by low pulmonary vascular resistance.

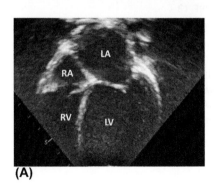

(A)

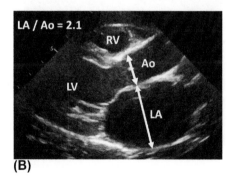

(B)

FIGURE 10

(A) Apical four-chamber view demonstrating severe left atrial and ventricular dilatation in a child with a large PDA. (B) The left atrial to aortic diameter ratio, determined from the parasternal long-axis view (*double arrows*), allows evaluation of the severity of left atrial dilatation. In this ratio, the aorta is used as a reference because, due to its rigidity, it does not dilate (unlike the left atrium) in response to left heart volume overload. Ratios exceeding 1.5:1, as in this example, are consistent with a hemodynamically significant shunt across the PDA. *Ao*, aorta; *LA*, left atrium; *LV*, left ventricle; *RA*, right atrium; *RV*, right ventricle.

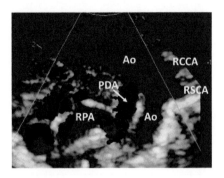

FIGURE 11

Suprasternal notch view in a patient with right aortic arch with mirror image branching and nonconfluent pulmonary arteries, independently supplied by bilateral arterial ducts. Note the presence of a right-sided PDA originating from the undersurface of the aortic arch and supplying the right pulmonary artery (left pulmonary artery not shown). *Ao*, aorta; *LCCA*, left common carotid artery; *LCCA*, left subclavian artery; *RPA*, right pulmonary artery.

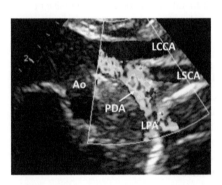

FIGURE 12

Same anomaly as in Figure 11 seen from a modified suprasternal notch view. Color flow mapping demonstrating a left-sided PDA arising from the base of the left subclavian artery, in continuity with the left pulmonary artery (right pulmonary artery not shown). *Ao*, aorta; *LCCA*, left common carotid artery; *LCCA*, left subclavian artery; *LPA*, left pulmonary artery.

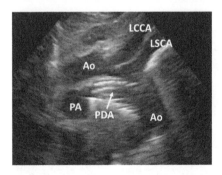

FIGURE 13

Ductal stenting is used as palliation in some patients with duct dependant pulmonary blood supply. Ductal stent visualized from the suprasternal notch view. *Ao*, aorta; *LCCA*, left common carotid artery; *LCCA*, left subclavian artery; *PA*, pulmonary artery.

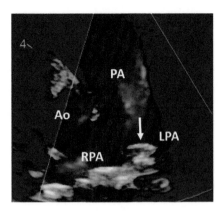

FIGURE 14

Zoomed parasternal short-axis view demonstrating a PDA occluder device (*arrow*) after transcatheter PDA closure. Color flow mapping showing no residual shunt across the device. *Ao*, aorta; *LPA*, left pulmonary artery; *PA*, pulmonary artery; *RPA*, right pulmonary artery.

Aorto-pulmonary window

Aorto-pulmonary window is a rare congenital malformation caused by an incomplete septation of the primitive arterial trunk in two separate great arteries. The pulmonary and aortic valves are not affected. Its hemodynamic consequences are very similar to those seen in PDA. Large defects, which are more common than small ones, usually lead to the early development of the symptoms of heart failure. In approximately half of the cases, this condition is associated with other cardiac anomalies that generally affect the outflow tracts. Treatment consists of either surgical or transcatheter closure of the defect.

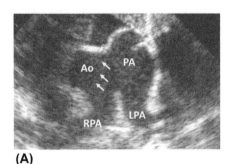
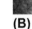

(A)   **(B)**

FIGURE 15

(A) Zoomed left subclavicular view illustrating a large aorto-pulmonary window. *Arrows* indicate the usual position of the aorto-pulmonary septum, absent in this view. (B) Small aorto-pulmonary window with a modest defect in the aorto-pulmonary septum (*arrow*). *Ao*, aorta; *LA*, left atrium; *LPA*, left pulmonary artery; *PA*, pulmonary artery; *RPA*, right pulmonary artery.

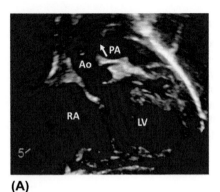 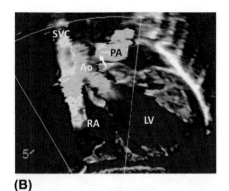

(A) **(B)**

FIGURE 16

(A) Subcostal long-axis view showing a large aorto-pulmonary window (*arrow*). (B) Color flow mapping illustrating turbulent blood flow between the aorta and the pulmonary artery (*arrow*). *Ao*, aorta; *LV*, left ventricle; *PA*, pulmonary artery; *RA*, right atrium; *SVC*, superior vena cava.

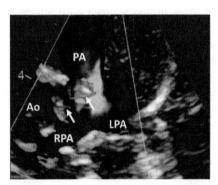

FIGURE 17

Zoomed parasternal short axis view in a patient with aorto-pulmonary window closed using a transcatheter approach. Note the presence of the occluder device. *Arrows* indicate the aortic and pulmonary discs anchoring the device. There is no residual shunt across the device detectable on color flow mapping. *Ao*, aorta; *LPA*, left pulmonary artery; *PA*, pulmonary artery; *RPA*, right pulmonary artery.

Coarctation of the aorta and interrupted aortic arch

17

Coarctation of the aorta

Coarctation of the aorta accounts for approximately 5%−10% of congenital heart defects and in many cases is diagnosed antenatally. The coarctation shelf typically develops at the level of the aortic isthmus opposite the insertion of the ductus arteriosus. The abdominal aorta is rarely affected. The spectrum of the disease ranges from critical to mild. Ductal closure in neonates with severe aortic narrowing generally precipitates a rapid clinical deterioration and cardiovascular collapse. On the other hand, the only manifestation in older patients with a mild degree of aortic obstruction may be isolated upper body hypertension.

Characteristic echocardiographic features include the presence of a localized luminal narrowing causing turbulent flow on color flow mapping. Systolic peaking with persistent forward diastolic flow produces a typical "saw-tooth" pattern on continuous wave Doppler. Nonpulsatile flow in the abdominal aorta is present in severe cases. The estimation of the transcoarctation pressure gradient may be unreliable in patients with cardiac dysfunction, large collaterals bypassing the obstruction or associated lesions such as aortic stenosis or ventricular septal defect with a left-to-right shunt.

Coarctation of the aorta often occurs together with other anomalies, including bicommissural (bicuspid) aortic valve, mitral valve dysplasia, hypoplastic left heart syndrome, or ventricular septal defect. It also frequently develops in patients with Turner syndrome. In young children, surgical resection is usually the treatment of choice, while in older patients transcatheter approach may be preferred. Despite successful initial intervention, recoarctation of the aorta develops in a minority of cases.

Atlas of Pediatric Echocardiography. https://doi.org/10.1016/B978-0-323-75981-6.00014-5

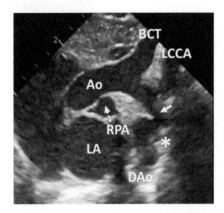

FIGURE 1

Suprasternal notch view showing a tapered distal transverse arch, hypoplastic aortic isthmus (*arrow*), and small posterior coarctation shelf (*asterisk*). Ao, aorta; BCT, brachiocephalic trunk; DAo, descending aorta; LA, left atrium; LCCA, left common carotid artery; RPA, right pulmonary artery.

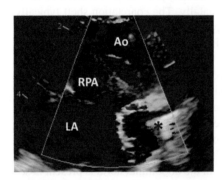

FIGURE 2

Tight coarctation of the aorta demonstrated from the suprasternal notch view. Color flow mapping showing turbulent flow starting at the level of the posterior shelf (*black asterisk*). Ao, aorta; LA, left atrium; RPA, right pulmonary artery.

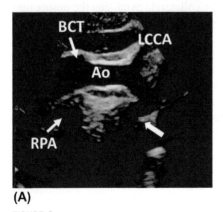

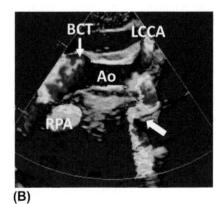

(A) **(B)**

FIGURE 3

(A) Coarctation of the aorta in a 5-week-old infant seen from the suprasternal notch view. *Arrow* indicates the posterior shelf, which significantly reduces the aortic luminal diameter. (B) Corresponding color flow mapping in the same patient. Note the absence of a ductus arteriosus. Ao, aorta; BCT, brachiocephalic trunk; LCCA, left common carotid artery; RPA, right pulmonary artery.

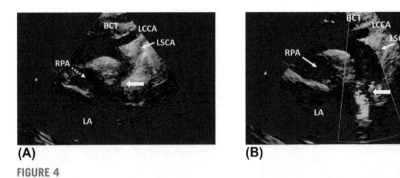

FIGURE 4

(A) Late diagnosis of aortic coarctation in a 3-year-old child with severe left ventricular dysfunction. Suprasternal notch view demonstrating gradual tapering of the aortic arch toward the coarctation site. The *arrow* denotes the posterior shelf. (B) Color flow mapping demonstrating significant flow acceleration caused by the posterior shelf (*arrow*). *BCT,* brachiocephalic trunk; *LA,* left atrium; *LCCA,* left common carotid artery; *LSCA,* left subclavian artery; *RPA,* right pulmonary artery.

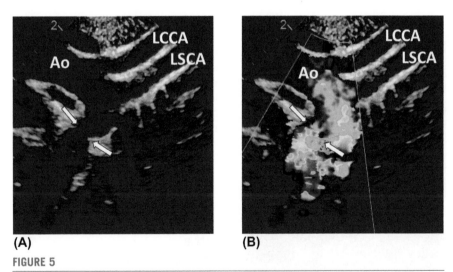

FIGURE 5

(A) Suprasternal notch view in a 4-year-old child with coarctation of the aorta. There is a circular (membranous) coarctation shelf distal to the left subclavian artery (*arrows*). (B) Turbulent flow across the coarctation site, as demonstrated by color flow mapping. *Ao,* aorta; *LCCA,* left common carotid artery; *LSCA,* left subclavian artery.

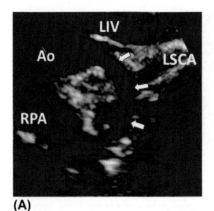

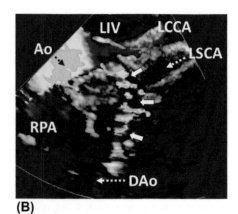

(A)   (B)

FIGURE 6

(A) Suprasternal notch view illustrating long segment hypoplasia of the aortic arch (*arrows*). (B) Color flow mapping showing turbulent flow across the affected segment. *Ao*, aorta; *DAo*, descending aorta; *LCCA*, left common carotid artery; *LIV*, left innominate vein; *LSCA*, left subclavian artery; *RPA*, right pulmonary artery.

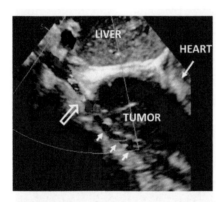

FIGURE 7

Subcostal view illustrating severe aortic narrowing caused by a thoracic tumor. The compression of the aorta starts in the midthoracic region (*small arrows*) and is most severe in the lower aspect of the tumor (*hollow arrow*).

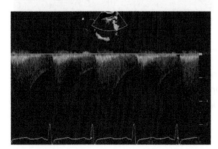

FIGURE 8

Continuous-wave Doppler of the descending thoracic aorta from the suprasternal notch view demonstrating increased blood flow velocity with systolic peaking and persistent forward diastolic flow. This produces a typical a "saw-tooth" pattern.

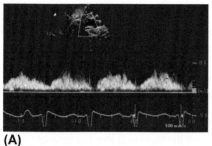 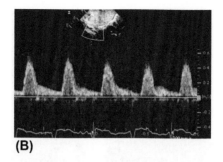

(A)   **(B)**

FIGURE 9

(A) Pulsed-wave Doppler of the abdominal aorta from the subcostal view in a child with severe aortic coarctation. The trace demonstrates low-velocity flow with nearly complete loss of pulsatility. (B) Same patient after successful surgical resection of the coarctation. The abdominal aorta pulse waveform normalizes.

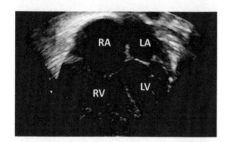

FIGURE 10

Apical four-chamber view demonstrating ventricular disproportion in a newborn with coarctation of the aorta. Note the severe right ventricular hypertrophy and dilatation, suggestive of significant pulmonary hypertension. The left ventricle is rather small, but apex forming. *LA*, left atrium; *LV*, left ventricle; *RA*, right atrium; *RV*, right ventricle.

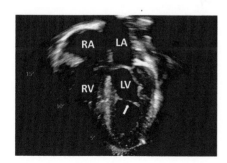

FIGURE 11

Late diagnosis of coarctation of the aorta in an older child. There is severe left ventricular hypertrophy due to increased ventricular afterload. Note the presence of a false ventricular tendon (*arrow*), which is often found in patients with coarctation of the aorta. *LA*, left atrium; *LV*, left ventricle; *RA*, right atrium; *RV*, right ventricle.

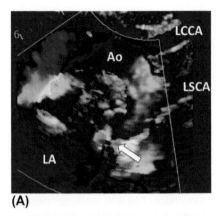

(A)

FIGURE 12

(A) Suprasternal notch view in a patient with late diagnosis of coarctation of the aorta. Note the turbulent flow starting at the level of the posterior shelf (*arrow*). (B) Same patient after successful implantation of a stent (*arrows*) across the affected segment. (C) Laminar blood flow across the stent indicates the optimal outcome of the intervention. *Ao*, aorta; *LA*, left atrium; *LCCA*, left common carotid artery; *LSCA*, left subclavian artery; *RPA*, right pulmonary artery.

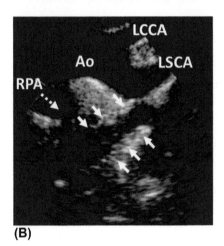

(B)

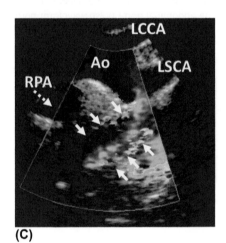

(C)

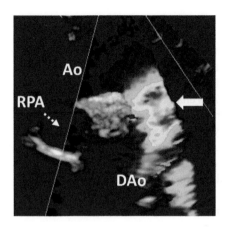

FIGURE 13

Suprasternal notch view with color flow mapping in a child after successful surgical resection of coarctation of the aorta. There is mildly turbulent flow (*arrow*) across the anastomosis site, but this is often the case even in patients with no residual pressure gradient between the upper and lower limbs. *Ao*, aorta; *DAo*, descending aorta; *RPA*, right pulmonary artery.

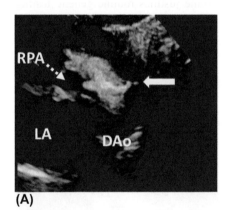

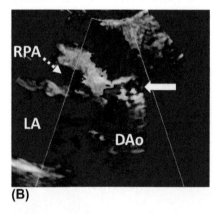

(A)   **(B)**

FIGURE 14

(A) Zoomed suprasternal notch view demonstrating recoarctation of the aorta, which developed several months after the initial surgical repair. The *arrows* indicate the narrowed anastomosis. (B) Color flow mapping in the same patient showing turbulent flow across the stenotic segment (*arrows*). *DAo*, descending aorta; *LA*, left atrium; *RPA*, right pulmonary artery.

Interrupted aortic arch

Interrupted aortic arch is a relatively uncommon duct dependant lesion, characterized by the absence of luminal continuity between the transverse arch and the proximal descending aorta. Depending on the location of the interruption site, three forms of the disease are distinguished. **Type A** is characterized by interruption distal to the left subclavian artery, **type B** by interruption between the left subclavian and the left common carotid artery, and **type C** by interruption between the left common carotid artery and the brachiocephalic trunk.

In almost all patients with an interrupted aortic arch, there is a posterior deviation of the infundibular septum, resulting in a malalignment ventricular septal defect and left ventricular outflow tract obstruction. It is thought that decreased aortic blood flow plays an important role in the development of aortic arch hypoplasia and interruption in utero.

Interrupted aortic arch often occurs together with persistent truncus arteriosus. Its frequent association with DiGeorge syndrome justifies routine genetic testing in affected patients. Cardiac surgery is the only treatment option and consists of aortic arch reconstruction.

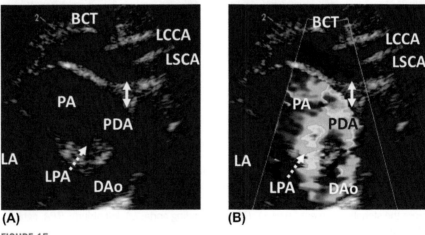

(A)   **(B)**

FIGURE 15

(A) Type A interrupted aortic arch seen from the suprasternal notch view. The interruption is distal to the left subclavian artery. The *double arrow* indicates the length of the interrupted segment. The descending aorta is in continuity with a widely open arterial duct. (B) Color flow mapping in the same patient. *BCT*, brachiocephalic trunk; *DAo*, descending aorta; *LA*, left atrium; *LCCA*, left common carotid artery; *LPA*, left pulmonary artery; *LSCA*, left subclavian artery; *PDA*, patent ductus arteriosus; *PA*, pulmonary artery.

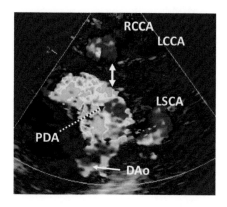

FIGURE 16

Suprasternal notch view demonstrating type B interrupted aortic arch in a newborn with persistent truncus arteriosus. The interrupted segment (*double arrow*) is between the left common carotid and the left subclavian artery. The right subclavian artery (not shown in this figure) arose from the descending aorta and had an aberrant course. *DAo*, descending aorta; *LCCA*, left common carotid artery; *LSCA*, left subclavian artery; *PDA*, patent ductus arteriosus; *RCCA*, right common carotid artery.

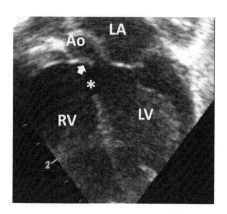

FIGURE 17

Apical five-chamber view in a newborn with an interrupted aortic arch. There is a posterior deviation of the infundibular septum, which is malaligned with the muscular septum. As a result, there is significant left ventricular outflow tract obstruction. The *asterisk* indicates an outlet ventricular septal defect. *Ao*, aorta; *LA*, left atrium; *LV*, left ventricle; *RV*, right ventricle.

Vascular rings

18

Vascular rings are congenital malformations characterized by tracheal and esophageal compression due to abnormalities of the great arteries, their branches and remnants. Based on the degree of encirclement of the trachea and the esophagus by these abnormal vessels, complete and incomplete vascular rings are distinguished.

Double aortic arch is the most common form of complete vascular ring. In this anomaly, both arches are usually patent, but atresia of one of the arches may be present. Right aortic arch with left ductus or ligamentum arteriosum represents another example of a complete vascular ring. Typically, this arrangement occurs in **right aortic arch with aberrant left subclavian artery** and **right aortic arch with mirror image branching**.

In the vast majority of cases, **left aortic arch with aberrant right subclavian artery** is associated with a left (and not a right) ductus or ligamentum arteriosum, thus forming an incomplete vascular ring only. **Left pulmonary artery sling** also falls into the category of incomplete vascular rings. The clinical picture in patients with vascular rings is variable and depends mainly on the severity of airway compression. In some children, the ring may be sufficiently loose not to cause any symptoms. In symptomatic patients, surgical division of the vascular ring is indicated.

Atlas of Pediatric Echocardiography. https://doi.org/10.1016/B978-0-323-75981-6.00034-0

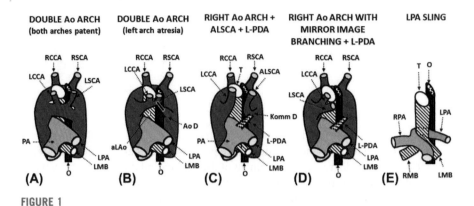

FIGURE 1

Common types of vascular rings. (A) Double aortic arch. Both arches are patent and have symmetric branching pattern. (B) Double aortic arch with atresia of the distal left arch. The black line indicates the atretic segment between the origin of the left subclavian artery and the tubular diverticulum arising from the descending aorta. Both the right and the incomplete left arch branch symmetrically. (C) Right aortic arch with aberrant left subclavian artery and left ductus or ligamentum arteriosum. The first branch of the aortic arch is the left common carotid artery. The left subclavian artery arises aberrantly as the last branch from a retroesophageal aortic diverticulum (Kommerell's diverticulum). The ring is closed by the left ligamentum arteriosum. (D) Right aortic arch with mirror image branching. As in the previous example, the ring is completed by the left ligamentum arteriosum. (E) In left pulmonary artery sling, the left pulmonary artery arises from the right pulmonary artery, thus encircling and compressing the distal trachea and the left main bronchus. *Ao D*, aortic diverticulum; *ALSCA*, aberrant left subclavian artery; *Komm D*, Kommerell's diverticulum; *LCCA*, left common carotid artery; *LMB*, left main bronchus; *LPA*, left pulmonary artery; *L-PDA*, left ductus or ligamentum arteriosum; *LSCA*, left subclavian artery; *O*, esophagus; *PA*, pulmonary artery; *RCCA*, right common carotid artery; *RMB*, right main bronchus; *RPA*, right pulmonary artery; *RSCA*, right subclavian artery; *T*, trachea.

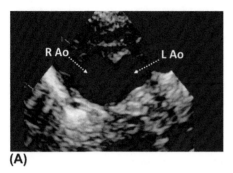 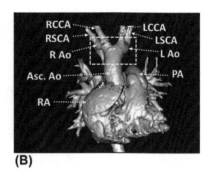

(A)   **(B)**

FIGURE 2

Double aortic arch. (A) Suprasternal notch view demonstrating the division of the ascending aorta into two aortic arches. (B) Corresponding CT picture. The dashed rectangle corresponds to the view shown in Figure 2A. *asc. Ao*, ascending aorta; *L Ao*, left aortic arch; *LCCA*, left common carotid artery; *LSCA*, left subclavian artery; *PA*, pulmonary artery; *RA*, right atrium; *R Ao*, right aortic arch; *RCCA*, right common carotid artery; *RSCA*, right subclavian artery.

(B) Courtesy of Dr. Oliver Tann.

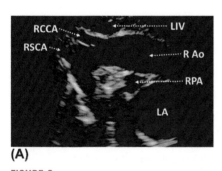 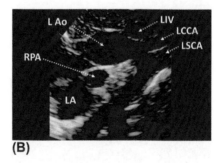

(A)   **(B)**

FIGURE 3

Suprasternal notch views in an infant with double aortic arch. Both arches are patent and similar in size. (A) Right aortic arch view. (B) Left aortic arch view. The subclavian and the common carotid arteries arise symmetrically from both arches. *LA*, left atrium; *L Ao*, left aortic arch; *LCCA*, left common carotid artery; *LIV*, left innominate vein; *LSCA*, left subclavian artery; *R Ao*, right aortic arch; *RCCA*, right common carotid artery; *RPA*, right pulmonary artery; *RSCA*, right subclavian artery.

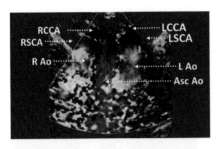

FIGURE 4

Double aortic arch seen from the suprasternal notch view. Note the division of the ascending aorta into the right and the left aortic arch, both have symmetric branching pattern. *Asc Ao*, ascending aorta; *L Ao*, left aortic arch; *LCCA*, left common carotid artery; *LSCA*, left subclavian artery; *R Ao*, right aortic arch; *RCCA*, right common carotid artery; *RSCA*, right subclavian artery.

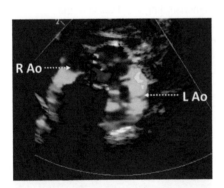

FIGURE 5

Double aortic arch seen from the suprasternal notch view. The left arch is larger than the right arch. *L Ao*, left aortic arch; *R Ao*, right aortic arch.

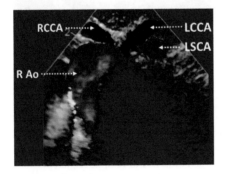

FIGURE 6

Suprasternal notch view demonstrating a double aortic arch with distal left arch atresia. Note the absence of flow between the left subclavian artery and the descending aorta. The right aortic arch is widely patent. In contrast to right aortic arch with mirror image branching, the branches arising from the right and the incomplete left arch have a more symmetric appearance. *LCCA*, left common carotid artery; *LSCA*, left subclavian artery; *R Ao*, right aortic arch; *RCCA*, right common carotid artery.

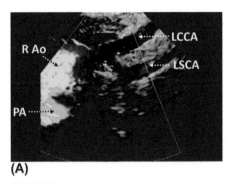 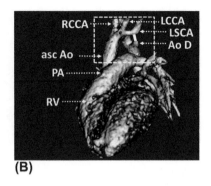

(A)   **(B)**

FIGURE 7

(A) Double aortic arch with distal left arch atresia. Zoomed suprasternal notch view showing branching of the incomplete left arch. No flow is detected between the left subclavian artery and the descending aorta. (B) Corresponding CT picture. The dashed rectangle corresponds to the view shown in Figure 7A. The atretic segment (white line) extends from the base of the left subclavian artery to the tubular diverticulum (not shown in Figure 7A), which arises from the descending aorta. *Ao D*, aortic diverticulum; *asc Ao*, ascending aorta; *LCCA*, left common carotid artery; *LSCA*, left subclavian artery; *PA*, pulmonary artery; *R Ao*, right aortic arch; *RCCA*, right common carotid artery; *RV*, right ventricle.

(B) Courtesy of Dr. Oliver Tann.

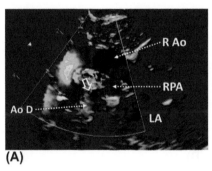 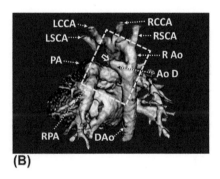

(A)   **(B)**

FIGURE 8

(A) Double aortic arch with distal left arch atresia. Suprasternal notch view showing the right aortic arch. The *hollow arrow* indicates a blind-ending tubular diverticulum arising from the descending aorta. The presence of this diverticulum helps to differentiate this anomaly from the right aortic arch with mirror image branching. (B) Corresponding CT picture (seen from behind). The dashed rectangle corresponds to the view shown in Figure 8A. The *hollow arrow* indicates the blind-ending aortic diverticulum. *Ao D*, aortic diverticulum; *DAo*, descending aorta; *LA*, left atrium; *LCCA*, left common carotid artery; *LSCA*, left subclavian artery *PA*, pulmonary artery; *R Ao*, right aortic arch; *RCCA*, right common carotid artery; *RPA*, right pulmonary artery; *RSCA*, right subclavian artery.

(B) Courtesy of Dr. Oliver Tann.

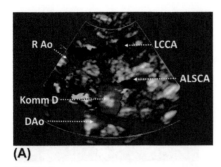
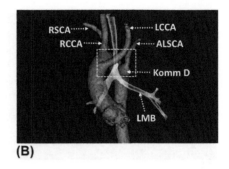

(A)   **(B)**

FIGURE 9

(A) Right aortic arch with aberrant left subclavian artery seen from the suprasternal notch view. The left common carotid artery is the first branch of the aortic arch and has a separate origin from the left subclavian artery. The latter arises aberrantly from an aneurysmal aortic diverticulum (Kommerell's diverticulum) and has a retroesophageal course. This is different from right aortic arch with a mirror branching, where both arteries have a common origin from the left brachiocephalic trunk. (B) Corresponding CT picture. The dashed rectangle corresponds to the view shown in Figure 9A. *ALSCA*, aberrant left subclavian artery; *DAo*, descending aorta; *Komm D*, Kommerell's diverticulum; *LCCA*, left common carotid artery; *LMB*, left main bronchus; *R Ao*, right aortic arch; *RCCA*, right common carotid artery; *RSCA*, right subclavian artery.

(B) Courtesy of Dr Oliver Tann.

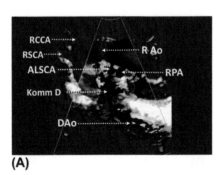
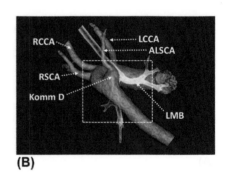

(A)   **(B)**

FIGURE 10

(A) Suprasternal notch view demonstrating right aortic arch with aberrant left subclavian artery. Note the origin of the aberrant left subclavian artery from the Kommerell's diverticulum. (B) Corresponding (rotated) CT picture. The dashed rectangle corresponds to the view shown in Figure 10A. *ALSCA*, aberrant left subclavian artery; *DAo*, descending aorta; *LMB*, left main bronchus; *R Ao*, right aortic arch; *RCCA*, right common carotid artery; *RPA*, right pulmonary artery; *RSCA*, right subclavian artery.

(B) Courtesy of Dr. Oliver Tann.

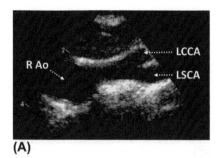 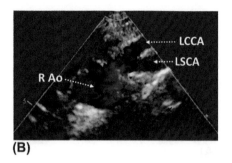

(A) **(B)**

FIGURE 11

(A) Suprasternal notch view demonstrating leftward branching of the brachiocephalic trunk in a patient with a right aortic arch with mirror image branching (see Chapter 1, Figure 30 for determination of the sidedness of the aortic arch). (B) Color flow mapping illustrating flow in the left brachiocephalic trunk, left common carotid artery, and left subclavian artery. *LCCA*, left common carotid artery; *LSCA*, left subclavian artery; *R Ao*, right aortic arch.

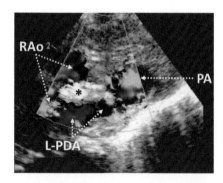

FIGURE 12

Suprasternal notch view (transverse plane) in an infant with a right aortic arch and a left ductus arteriosus. The ductus arteriosus has a retroesophageal course and encircles the trachea (*asterisk*) and the esophagus. The trachea has a hyperechogenic appearance. *L-PDA*, left ductus arteriosum; *PA*, pulmonary artery; *R Ao*, right aortic arch.

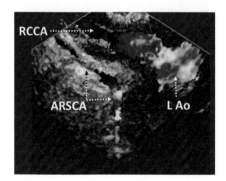

FIGURE 13

Left aortic arch with aberrant right subclavian artery visualized from the suprasternal notch view. The first branch originating from the aortic arch is the right common carotid artery. Note the separate origin of the right subclavian artery, which arises aberrantly from the distal part of the aortic arch. *ARSCA*, right subclavian artery; *L Ao*, left aortic arch; *RCCA*, right common carotid artery.

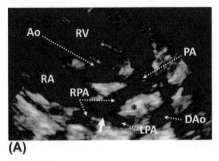 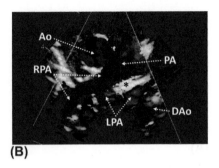

(A) **(B)**

FIGURE 14

(A) Left pulmonary artery sling visualized from the parasternal short-axis view. The left pulmonary artery arises from the right pulmonary artery (*arrow*) and encircles the distal trachea (*asterisk*) and the left main bronchus. (B) Color flow mapping demonstrating blood flow in the pulmonary artery and pulmonary artery branches. *Ao*, aorta; *DAo*, descending aorta; *LPA*, left pulmonary artery; *PA*, pulmonary artery; *RA*, right atrium; *RPA*, right pulmonary artery; *RV*, right ventricle.

Pulmonary and systemic venous anomalies

19

Disorders resulting from abnormal development of the pulmonary and systemic veins include a number of conditions with different clinical symptomatology. Some of them are benign and do not necessitate any treatment, while others, such as an obstructed total anomalous pulmonary venous connection, can cause critical illness, requiring an early cardiac intervention. Echocardiography plays an important role in the diagnosis of these anomalies.

Pulmonary venous anomalies

The early phase of pulmonary venous development is characterized by drainage of the pulmonary vascular bed into the cardinal veins, from which the systemic venous circulation is later derived. These pulmonary to systemic venous connections regress with the formation of the common pulmonary vein, connecting the pulmonary vascular bed to the left atrium. However, if this regression is incomplete, the connection between the pulmonary and systemic veins may persist, resulting in an anomalous pulmonary venous connection.

In **total anomalous pulmonary venous connection (TAPVC)**, there is no connection between the pulmonary veins and the left atrium, while in **partial anomalous pulmonary venous connection (PAPVC)**, at least one pulmonary vein is connected to the left atrium. Different types of TAPVC are summarized in Figure 1.

Cor triatriatum sinister is a rare cardiac defect in which the left atrium is divided by a membrane into two separate chambers. In some cases, the membrane causes obstruction to blood flow. It is thought that this condition is the result of an anomalous incorporation of the common pulmonary vein into the left atrium during the development of the heart. **Pulmonary vein stenosis** is an infrequent anomaly that is either congenital or acquired (most often after previous surgery on pulmonary veins). It usually carries a poor prognosis.

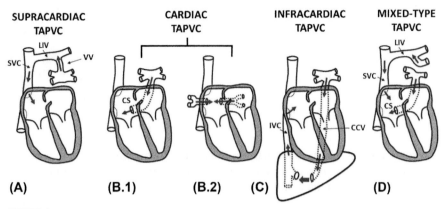

(A)   **(B.1)**   **(B.2)**   **(C)**   **(D)**

FIGURE 1

Types of TAPVC. (A) Example of **supracardiac TAPVC** in which the pulmonary venous confluence drains via an ascending vertical vein (VV) into the left innominate vein (LIV). (B) Examples of **cardiac TAPVC**: (1) the pulmonary venous confluence drains into the coronary sinus (CS); (2) the confluence of the right and left-sided pulmonary veins drain separately into the right atrium. (C) **Infracardiac TAPVC** with the pulmonary venous confluence draining via a common collector vein (CCV) into either the portal vein, the hepatic vein, or the inferior vena cava (IVC). (D) Example of **mixed type TAPVC** in which the right upper pulmonary vein drains into the left innominate vein. The confluence of the remaining pulmonary veins drains into the coronary sinus.

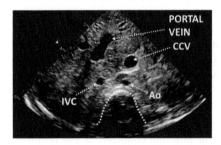

FIGURE 2

Subcostal (situs) view illustrating the infradiaphragmatic portion of the common collector vein in a patient with infracardiac TAPVC. There is portal vein dilatation due to the common collector vein joining the portal venous system. *Dotted line* indicates the spine. *Ao*, aorta; *CCV*, common collector vein; *IVC*, inferior vena cava.

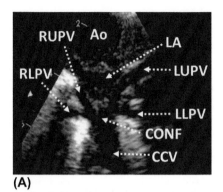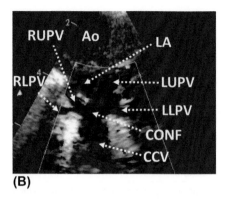

(A)   **(B)**

FIGURE 3

(A) Suprasternal notch view (frontal plane) demonstrating union of the right- and left-sided pulmonary veins into a common confluence, giving rise to the common collector vein. (B) Color flow mapping showing a downward flow in the common collector vein. *Ao*, aorta; *CONF*, confluence; *CCV*, common collector vein; *LA*, left atrium; *LLPV*, left lower pulmonary vein; *LUPV*, left upper pulmonary vein; *RLPV*, right lower pulmonary vein; *RUPV*, right upper pulmonary vein.

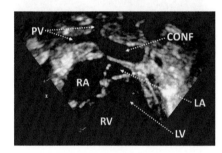

FIGURE 4

Zoomed apical four-chamber view in a child with infradiaphragmatic TAPVC. The pulmonary veins join into a common confluence behind the left atrium. Note the absence of connection between the confluence and the left atrium. *CONF*, confluence; *LA*, left atrium; *LV*, left ventricle; *PV*, pulmonary veins; *RA*, right atrium; *RV*, right ventricle.

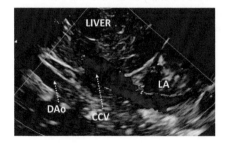

FIGURE 5

Infradiaphragmatic TAPVC. Subcostal view (sagittal plane) illustrating the course of the common collector vein, starting posterior to the left atrium, then crossing the diaphragm. *CCV*, common collector vein; *DAo*, descending aorta; *LA*, left atrium.

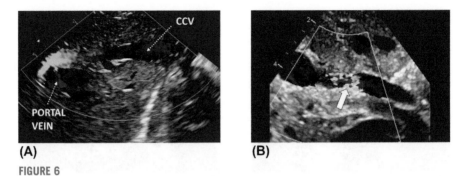

FIGURE 6

Infradiaphragmatic TAPVC. (A) Subcostal view (transverse plane) showing the course of the common collector vein, joining the portal venous system. (B) Intrahepatic obstruction to pulmonary venous flow (*arrow*), as demonstrated on color flow mapping. *CCV*, common collector vein.

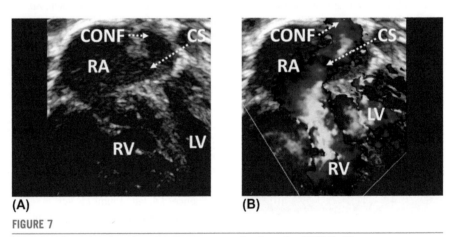

FIGURE 7

(A) Apical four-chamber view showing an example of cardiac TAPVC. The common confluence of the pulmonary veins is connected to the coronary sinus, draining into the right atrium. (B) Color flow mapping showing blood flow from the confluence into the right atrium via the coronary sinus. *CONF*, confluence; *CS*, coronary sinus; *LV*, left ventricle; *RA*, right atrium; *RV*, right ventricle.

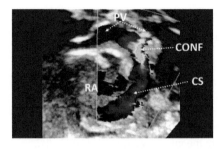

FIGURE 8

Zoomed subcostal view in a child with cardiac TAPVC. The right and left pulmonary veins join in a common confluence, which is in continuity with the coronary sinus, draining into the right atrium ("whale tail" sign). *CONF*, confluence; *CS*, coronary sinus; *PV*, right and left-sided pulmonary veins; *RA*, right atrium.

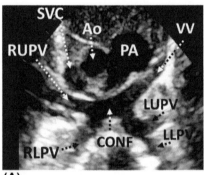

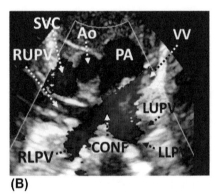

(A)   **(B)**

FIGURE 9

Supracardiac TAPVC. (A) Suprasternal notch view (frontal plane) showing the formation of a common confluence of the right and left-sided pulmonary veins. The confluence is connected to the systemic venous circulation via an ascending vertical vein. (B) Color flow mapping demonstrating upward flow in the vertical vein. *Ao*, aorta; *CONF*, confluence; *LLPV*, left lower pulmonary vein; *LUPV*, left upper pulmonary vein; *PA*, pulmonary artery; *RLPV*, right lower pulmonary vein; *RUPV*, right upper pulmonary vein; *SVC*, superior vena cava; *VV*, vertical vein.

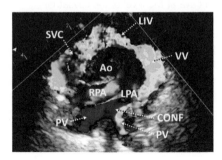

FIGURE 10

Suprasternal notch view (frontal plane) in an infant with supracardiac TAPVC. The right- and left-sided pulmonary veins join in a common confluence, which drains via an ascending vertical vein into the left innominate vein. As a result, the superior vena cava is dilated and there is generous flow in it. *Ao*, aorta; *CONF*, confluence; *LIV*, left innominate vein; *LPA*, left pulmonary artery; *PV*, right- and left-sided pulmonary veins; *RPA*, right pulmonary artery; *SVC*, superior vena cava; *VV*, vertical vein.

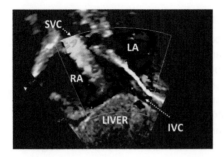

FIGURE 11

Subcostal (bicaval) short-axis view in a child with supracardiac TAPVC. Color flow mapping illustrating disproportionate venous return from caval veins. There is an abundance of flow from the superior vena cava due to the vertical vein draining into its territory. Note significantly less flow from the inferior vena cava. TAPVC. *IVC*, inferior vena cava; *LA*, left atrium; *RA*, right atrium; *SVC*, superior vena cava.

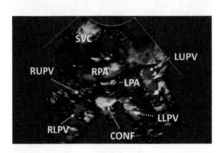

FIGURE 12

Mixed type TAPVC seen from the suprasternal notch view (frontal plane). The left lower and the right-sided pulmonary veins form a common confluence, draining into the coronary sinus (not shown). The left upper pulmonary vein has an upward course and drains separately into the left innominate vein (not shown). *CONF*, confluence; *LLPV*, left lower pulmonary vein; *LPA*, left pulmonary artery; *LUPV*, left upper pulmonary vein; *RLPV*, right lower pulmonary vein; *RPA*, right pulmonary artery; *RUPV*, right upper pulmonary vein; *SVC*, superior vena cava.

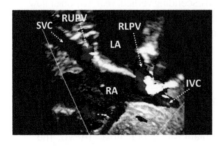

FIGURE 13

PAPVC seen from the subcostal (bicaval) short-axis view. The right upper pulmonary vein drains into the superior vena cava at the level of the cavoatrial junction. Similarly, the right lower pulmonary vein connects to the junction between the inferior vena cava and the right atrium. There was normal drainage of the left-sided pulmonary veins (not shown). *SVC*, superior vena cava; *IVC*, inferior vena cava; *RA*, right atrium; *LA*, left atrium; *RUPV*, right upper pulmonary vein; *RLPV*, right lower pulmonary vein.

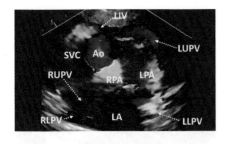

FIGURE 14

Suprasternal notch view (frontal plane) with color flow mapping showing anomalous drainage of the left upper pulmonary vein into the left innominate vein. The remaining pulmonary veins drain normally into the left atrium. *Ao*, aorta; *LA*, left atrium; *LLPV*, left lower pulmonary vein; *LPA*, left pulmonary artery; *LUPV*, left upper pulmonary vein; *RLPV*, right lower pulmonary vein; *RPA*, right pulmonary artery; *RUPV*, right upper pulmonary vein; *SVC*, superior vena cava.

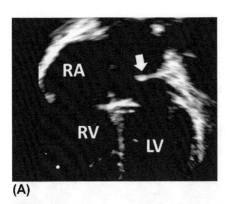

(A)

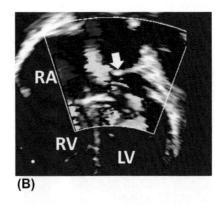

(B)

FIGURE 15

(A) Zoomed apical four-chamber view in a child with cor triatriatum sinister. The *arrow* indicates a membrane that partially divides the left atrium into two separate chambers. (B) Color flow mapping demonstrating mild flow turbulence caused by the membrane. *LV*, left ventricle; *RA*, right atrium; *RV*, right ventricle.

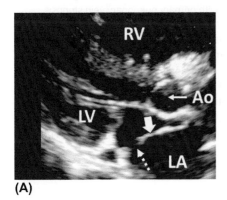

(A)

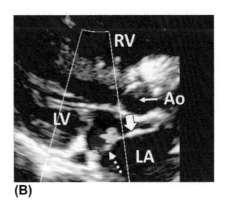

(B)

FIGURE 16

(A) Cor triatriatum sinister seen from the parasternal long-axis view. The left atrium is divided by a membrane (*arrow*), which has a small foramen (*dotted arrow*) in the lower aspect. (B) Color flow mapping demonstrating flow turbulence starting at the level of the foramen. *Ao*, aorta; *LA*, left atrium; *LV*, left ventricle; *RV*, right ventricle.

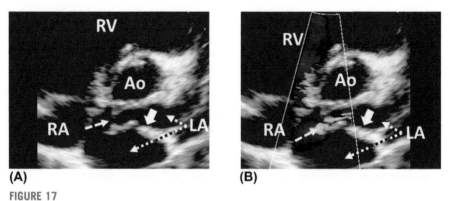

(A)   **(B)**

FIGURE 17

(A) Zoomed parasternal short axis view in a child with cor triatriatum sinister. The left atrium is incompletely divided by a membrane (*arrow*) into two compartments, which communicate with each other through a small foramen (*dashed arrow*). (B) The foramen is restrictive and causes obstruction to blood flow, as demonstrated on color flow mapping. *Ao*, aorta; *LA*, left atrium; *RA*, right atrium; *RV*, right ventricle.

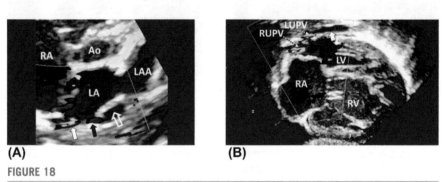

(A)   **(B)**

FIGURE 18

(A) Zoomed parasternal short-axis view in a child with primary pulmonary vein stenosis. There is a severe focal narrowing of the right (*white arrow*) and left (*black arrow*) pulmonary veins as they enter the left atrium. *Hollow arrow* indicates prestenotic dilatation of the left upper pulmonary vein. (B) Same heart seen from the subcostal four-chamber view. Color flow mapping demonstrating turbulent flow across the distal segment of the right and left upper pulmonary veins. There is left upper pulmonary vein dilatation (*arrow*) proximal to the stenosis. Note significant right atrial and ventricular dilatation consistent with severe pulmonary hypertension. *Ao*, aorta; *LA*, left atrium; *LAA*, left atrial appendage; *LUPV*, left upper pulmonary vein; *LV*, left ventricle; *RA*, right atrium; *RUPV*, right upper pulmonary vein; *RV*, right ventricle.

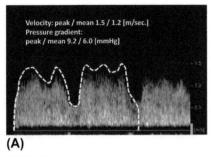 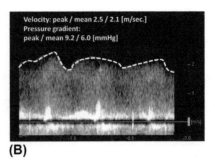

(A) **(B)**

FIGURE 19

Continuous-wave Doppler of the right upper pulmonary vein in a child with primary pulmonary vein stenosis. (A) Early in the disease, the pulmonary venous flow is phasic, but does not return not to the baseline. The peak velocity is increased. (B) The flow becomes continuous with the progression of the disease. There is a further increase in the stenotic gradient.

Systemic venous anomalies

The persistence of the **left superior vena cava** (LSVC) draining into the coronary sinus is the most common systemic venous anomaly. Despite its frequent association with various cardiac malformations, it is considered a normal variant if found in isolation. Most patients with LSVC have bilateral superior venae cavae, but in some cases, only the LSVC persists.

Levoatrial cardinal vein is an anomalous connection between the left atrium and usually the right superior vena cava (SVC) or the left innominate vein. It represents an embryological connection between the pulmonary vascular bed and the cardinal venous system, from which the systemic veins are derived. The presence of the levoatrial cardinal vein is often associated with left-sided obstructive lesions, such as mitral stenosis, where it decompresses the left atrium. **Interruption of the inferior vena cava** is typically present in left atrial isomerism, where blood from the lower body is drained into the SVC via the azygos (or hemi-azygos) venous system (azygos or hemi-azygos continuation).

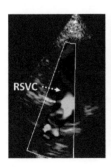 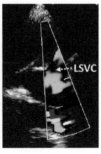

FIGURE 20

Suprasternal notch view (frontal plane) demonstrating bilateral superior venae cavae in a patient after bilateral cavo-pulmonary connections. *LSVC*, superior vena cava; *RSVC*, superior vena cava.

Courtesy of Prof Jan Marek.

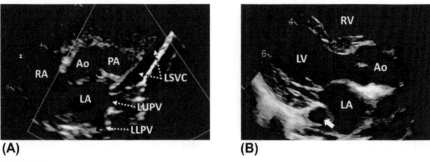

FIGURE 21

(A) Suprasternal notch view (frontal plane) demonstrating the left superior vena cava extending down to the lateral aspect of the left atrium (its connection to the coronary sinus is not shown). (B) Parasternal long-axis view illustrating dilatation of the coronary sinus (*arrow*) due to drainage of the left superior vena cava into it. *Ao*, aorta; *LA*, left atrium; *LLPV*, left lower pulmonary vein; *LSVC*, superior vena cava; *LUPV*, left upper pulmonary vein; *LV*, left ventricle; *PA*, pulmonary artery; *RA*, right atrium; *RV*, right ventricle.

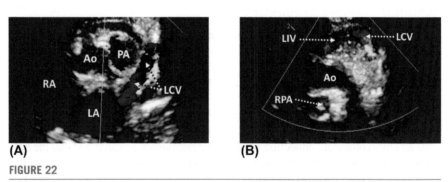

FIGURE 22

(A) Suprasternal notch view (frontal plane) demonstrating the levoatrial cardinal vein connecting to the roof of the left atrium. There is an upward flow in the vessel. (B) Modified suprasternal notch view showing the distal end of the same levoatrial cardinal vein connecting to the left innominate vein. *Ao*, aorta; *LA*, left atrium; *LCV*, levoatrial cardinal vein; *LIV*, left innominate vein; *PA*, pulmonary artery; *RA*, right atrium; *RPA*, right pulmonary artery.

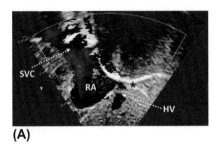
(A)

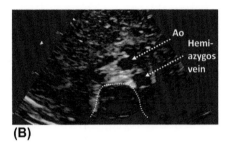
(B)

FIGURE 23

(A) Child with left atrial isomerism and interrupted inferior vena cava. Subcostal (bicaval) short-axis view showing venous return from the superior vena cava and hepatic veins only. No flow from the inferior vena cava can be demonstrated. The *black asterisk* indicates the usual location of the inferior vena cava in a normal individual. (B) Same patient. Subcostal transverse (situs) view illustrating a dilated hemi-azygos vein draining blood from the lower body (hemi-azygos continuation). *Dotted line* represents the spine. *Ao,* aorta; *HV,* hepatic vein; *RA,* right atrium; *SVC,* superior vena cava.

Congenital coronary artery abnormalities

20

Congenital coronary artery abnormalities are often difficult to diagnose on echocardiography due to the size of the coronary arteries, especially in small children. Patients with **anomalous left coronary artery from the pulmonary artery (ALCAPA)** usually present early in life with symptoms of severe heart failure. This is caused by a postnatal decrease in pulmonary pressure leading to flow reversal in the left coronary artery and myocardial ischemia. The term **coronary artery fistula** refers to an abnormal connection between a coronary artery and a cardiac chamber or less commonly a great vessel. In many patients, the feeding coronary artery is significantly dilated and has a tortuous course. The most common are isolated fistulas draining into the right heart chambers.

Abnormalities of coronary artery origin from the aorta can occur either in isolation or in association with other heart defects (mainly tetralogy of Fallot and transposition of the great arteries). Their presence is often revealed by a syncopal event induced by physical activity. However, in many patients, the diagnosis of anomalous coronary artery origin from the aorta is an incidental finding. The treatment of congenital coronary artery abnormalities depends on the type of the lesion. In some cases, it consists in avoidance of exercise, while in others surgical or interventional therapy is required. Kawasaki disease is a major cause of acquired coronary artery disease in childhood and is discussed separately in Chapter 23.

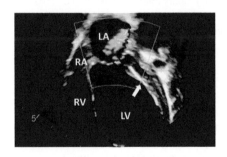

FIGURE 1

Apical four-chamber view demonstrating the typical left ventricular appearance in ALCAPA. The left ventricle is severely dysfunctional, and there is aneurysmal dilatation of the apex. Note the increased echo brightness of the antero-lateral papillary muscle (*arrow*) and the surrounding myocardium, which is caused by ischemia. Color flow mapping showing significant mitral regurgitation. *LA*, left atrium; *LV*, left ventricle; *RA*, right atrium; *RV*, right ventricle.

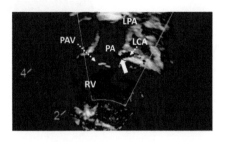

FIGURE 2

Zoomed apical view illustrating the right ventricular outflow tract in a child with ALCAPA. *White arrow* denotes the origin of the left coronary artery from the pulmonary artery. Color flow mapping showing retrograde coronary flow to the pulmonary artery. *LCA*, left coronary artery; *LPA*, left pulmonary artery; *PA*, pulmonary artery; *PAV*, pulmonary valve; *RV*, right ventricle.

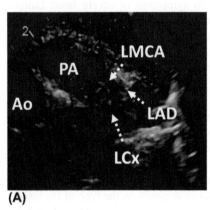
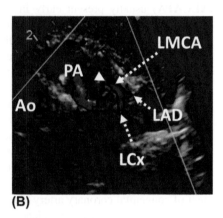

(A) **(B)**

FIGURE 3

(A) Zoomed high parasternal short-axis view in a child with ALCAPA. The left coronary artery arises from the lateral aspect of the pulmonary artery and is distant from the aorta. (B) Note the retrograde coronary blood flow to the pulmonary artery as illustrated on color flow mapping. *Ao*, aorta; *LCx*, left circumflex coronary artery; *LAD*, left anterior descending coronary artery; *LMCA*, left main coronary artery.

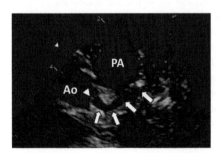

FIGURE 4

Zoomed high parasternal short-axis view in a child with ALCAPA. The *arrows* indicate the course of the left coronary artery, the origin of which is separated from the aorta (arrowhead). The connection between the left coronary artery and the pulmonary artery is not shown in this figure. *Ao*, aorta; *PA*, pulmonary artery.

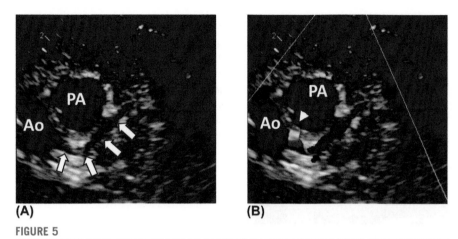

FIGURE 5

(A) Zoomed high parasternal short-axis view in a patient with ALCAPA. *Arrows* indicate the course of the left coronary artery that wrongly appears to originate from the aorta (Ao). (B) Color flow mapping in the same patient showing retrograde flow in the left coronary artery and its true origin from the pulmonary artery (PA) (arrowhead). In light of the above, the origin of the left coronary artery should only be considered as normal if there is antegrade flow in it.

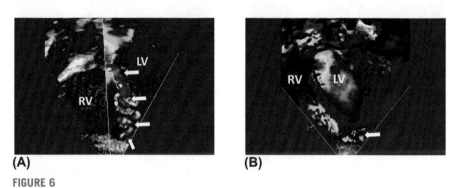

FIGURE 6

(A) Zoomed apical view in a patient with a large coronary fistula from the left anterior descending coronary artery to the right ventricle. The coronary artery is significantly dilated and has a tortuous course (*arrows*). (B) More posterior view in the same patient demonstrating the exit point of the fistula into the apical portion of the right ventricle. *LV*, left ventricle; *RV*, right ventricle.

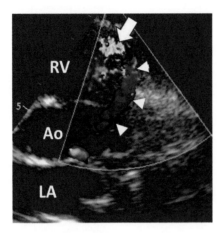

FIGURE 7

Parasternal short-axis view demonstrating a large coronary fistula connecting the left anterior descending coronary artery (*arrowheads*) to the outlet portion of the right ventricle (*arrow*). Color flow mapping showing generous coronary flow. *Ao*, aorta; *LA*, left atrium; *RV*, right ventricle.

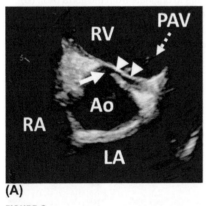

(A)

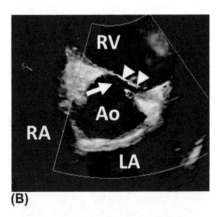

(B)

FIGURE 8

(A) Zoomed parasternal short-axis view in a patient with previous exertional syncope. Note the anomalous origin of the left main coronary artery from the right coronary cusp (*arrow*). The origin is central, away from the commissural junction. The left main coronary artery passes obliquely between the aorta and the pulmonary artery and appears narrowed in its proximal interarterial course (*arrowheads*). (B) Coronary blood flow demonstrated on color flow mapping. *Ao*, aorta; *LA*, left atrium; *PAV*, pulmonary valve; *RA*, right atrium; *RV*, right ventricle.

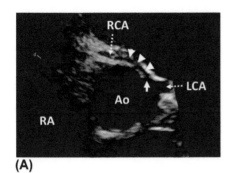
(A)

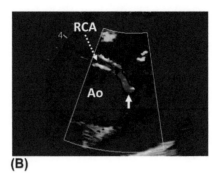
(B)

FIGURE 9

(A) Parasternal short-axis view illustrating anomalous right coronary artery origin (*arrow*) from the left coronary sinus, close to the commissure between the left and right coronary cusp. The origin is adjacent but separate from the left main coronary artery origin. The proximal right coronary artery is narrowed (*arrowheads*) as it courses between the aorta and the right ventricular outflow tract. (B) Same anomaly in a different patient. Right coronary artery flow demonstrated on color flow mapping. *Arrow* indicates the juxta-commissural origin of the right coronary artery. *Ao*, aorta; *LCA*, left coronary artery; *RA*, right atrium.

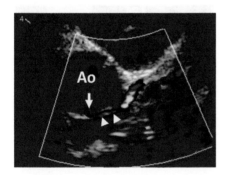

FIGURE 10

Zoomed parasternal short-axis view in a child with juxta-commissural origin of the left coronary artery from noncoronary sinus (*arrow*). The vessel is narrowed proximally (*arrowheads*). *Ao*, aorta.

Courtesy of Professor Jan Marek.

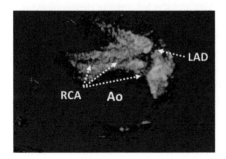

FIGURE 11

Zoomed parasternal short-axis view. Left anterior descending coronary artery (LAD) arising from the right coronary artery (RCA) in a patient with tetralogy of Fallot. Due to the LAD crossing the right ventricular outflow tract, surgical repair with transannular patch is not possible in this child.

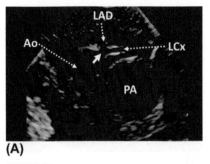
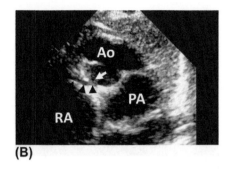

(A)   **(B)**

FIGURE 12

Detailed examination of the coronary artery anatomy in patients with transposition of the great arteries (TGA) plays an important role in preparation for the arterial switch operation. By convention, when "looking" from the nonfacing aortic sinus, the right-hand facing sinus refers to sinus 1 and the left-hand facing sinus to sinus 2. (A) Parasternal short-axis view illustrating normal coronary artery arrangement in TGA. The left main coronary artery originates from sinus 1 and bifurcates into the left anterior descending coronary artery (LAD) and the left circumflex coronary artery (LCx). (B) The right coronary artery (*arrowheads*) arises from sinus 2 (*arrow*). *PA*, pulmonary artery; *RA*, right atrium.

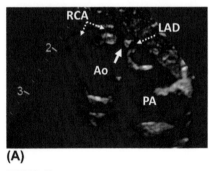
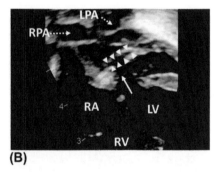

(A)   **(B)**

FIGURE 13

(A) Infant with transposition of the great arteries. Zoomed high parasternal short-axis view showing a common origin of the right coronary artery and the left anterior descending coronary artery from sinus 1. The left circumflex coronary artery originated from sinus 2 (not shown). (B) Same heart seen from a zoomed subcostal four-chamber view. The *arrowheads* delineate the left circumflex coronary artery coursing posterior to the pulmonary artery. The *white arrow* indicates the orientation of the left ventricular outflow tract. *Ao* aorta; *LPA*, left pulmonary artery; *LV*, left ventricle; *PA*, pulmonary artery; *RA*, right atrium; *RPA*, right pulmonary artery; *RV*, right ventricle.

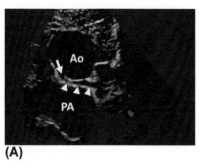
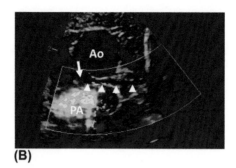

(A)   **(B)**

FIGURE 14

(A) Zoomed high parasternal short-axis view in a child with ventriculo-arterial discordance and antero-posterior relationship of the great arteries. The *arrow* indicates a juxta-commissural origin of the left coronary artery (*arrowheads*) from sinus 2 at an acute angle. The vessel has an intramural course. (B) Coronary blood flow demonstrated on color flow mapping. *Ao*, aorta; *PA*, pulmonary artery.

Acquired heart diseases and other conditions

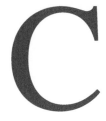

Myocarditis

21

Myocarditis is an inflammation of the myocardium that is most often caused by viruses. Bacterial, fungal, or noninfectious etiology is also possible. The inflammatory process is a complex cascade of chronological events that can lead to a fulminant clinical picture or progress to a more chronic phase. There is emerging evidence that myocarditis plays a fundamental role in the pathogenesis of some cases of dilated cardiomyopathy.

The inflammation may affect the heart muscle in a diffuse or focal fashion, leading to global or regional dysfunction. The focal process is often difficult to detect and may be missed even on endomyocardial biopsy. Echocardiographic diagnosis of myocarditis is based on the presence of some nonspecific features, including pericardial effusion, myocardial edema, systolic or diastolic dysfunction, ventricular dilatation, or new valvar regurgitation. However, some patients with milder forms of the disease may have a normal echocardiogram despite evidence of myocarditis on some other imaging modalities.

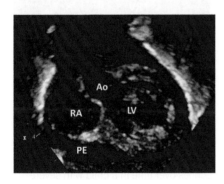

FIGURE 1

Subcostal long-axis view in a patient with myocarditis and global systolic dysfunction. Note the presence of diffuse left ventricular edema and a small pericardial effusion. *Ao,* aorta; *LV,* left ventricle; *RA,* right atrium; *PE,* pericardial effusion.

Atlas of Pediatric Echocardiography. https://doi.org/10.1016/B978-0-323-75981-6.00007-8
Copyright © 2021 Elsevier Inc. All rights reserved.

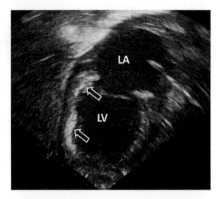

FIGURE 2

Apical two-chamber view in a child with myocarditis demonstrating widespread inflammatory infiltrate affecting the inferior segments (*hollow arrows*). *LA*, left atrium; *LV*, left ventricle.

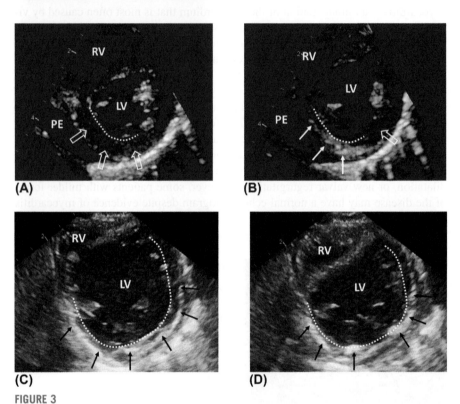

FIGURE 3

Parasternal short-axis views showing the series of echoes over time in a child with severe myocarditis. (A) The disease starts with myocardial swelling of the inferior and to some extent the lateral segments (*hollow arrows*). The affected segments are hypoechogenic and appear thickened due to edema. The dotted line indicates the hypokinetic segments. Note the presence of a pericardial effusion. (B) As the disease progresses, a hyperechogenic inflammatory infiltrate develops in the above-mentioned segments (*white arrows*). Myocardial edema then progresses to the lateral segments (*hollow arrow*), which also become dysfunctional (*dotted line*). (C and D) After some time, the inflammatory infiltrate extensively affects the infero-lateral segments (*black arrows*). The areas of significantly increased echo brightness are suggestive of myocardial necrosis.
(C) represents a diastolic frame, (D) a systolic frame. When compared, it is apparent that there is only a contraction of the interventricular septum. The *dotted line* indicates severely hypokinetic to akinetic segments. *LV*, left ventricle; *RV*, right ventricle.

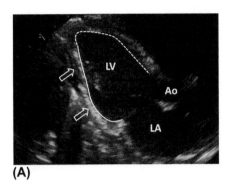 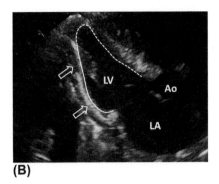

(A) **(B)**

FIGURE 4

(A, B) Parasternal long-axis view in a child with myocarditis. There is an extensive inflammatory infiltrate affecting the posterior segments (*hollow arrows*) that are akinetic (*solid line*). Comparison between the diastolic (A) and systolic (B) frames shows contraction limited to the septal segments only (*dashed line*). *LA*, left atrium; *LV*, left ventricle; Ao aorta.

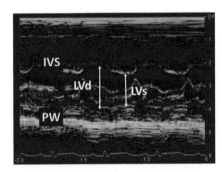

FIGURE 5

Patient with myocarditis and dysfunction of the posterior wall of the left ventricle. Parasternal long-axis M-mode showing significant hypokinesia of the posterior wall. There is good contractility of the interventricular septum. *IVS*, interventricular septum; *LVd*, left ventricular end-diastolic diameter; *LVs*, left ventricular end-systolic diameter; *PW*, posterior wall.

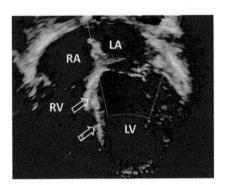

FIGURE 6

Apical four-chamber view in a child with myocarditis. The *hollow arrows* indicate the hyperechogenicity of the interventricular septum consistent with an inflammatory infiltrate. The left ventricle is dilated and dysfunctional and as a result there is mitral regurgitation. *LA*, left atrium; *LV*, left ventricle; *RA*, right atrium; *RV*, right ventricle.

Cardiomyopathies

22

Cardiomyopathy is an umbrella term for a group of myocardial disorders characterized by a structural and functional abnormality of the heart muscle, which is not secondary to other causes such as hypertension, congenital heart disease, valvar disease, or coronary artery disease. Based on morphological and functional features, cardiomyopathies can be divided into subtypes, including in particular **dilated**, **hypertrophic**, and **restrictive cardiomyopathy**. **Noncompaction cardiomyopathy** should be mentioned as a rare form of heart muscle disease.

Recent advances in understanding the genetic nature of cardiomyopathies have made it possible to identify causative genetic mutations, especially in patients who are affected by a familial form of the disease. In light of this, echocardiographic screening plays an important role in the detection of affected family members.

Cardiomyopathies in children may manifest very early in life and could cause significant morbidity and mortality. Despite limited options, early detection and appropriate treatment may improve outcomes.

Dilated cardiomyopathy

A characteristic feature of dilated cardiomyopathy (DCM) is the presence of left ventricular systolic dysfunction and dilatation that is not due to other secondary causes. Left ventricular diastolic dysfunction and right ventricular dysfunction or dilatation may also be present but they are not part of the diagnostic criteria. It has become increasingly evident that there is an overlap between viral myocarditis and later progression to dilated cardiomyopathy. Familial genetic forms of DCM appear to account for approximately one-quarter of cases, predominantly with an autosomal dominant pattern.

Atlas of Pediatric Echocardiography. https://doi.org/10.1016/B978-0-323-75981-6.00013-3

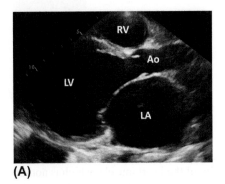
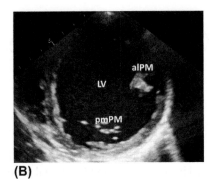

(A) **(B)**

FIGURE 1

(A) Parasternal long short-axis view in a patient with DCM. The left ventricle is significantly dilated and the myocardium has a thin-walled appearance due to stretching. There is also severe left atrial dilatation. (B) Same heart seen from the parasternal short-axis view. *alPM*, antero-lateral papillary muscle; *Ao*, aorta; *LA*, left atrium; *LV*, left ventricle; *pmPM*, postero-medial papillary muscle; *RV*, right ventricle.

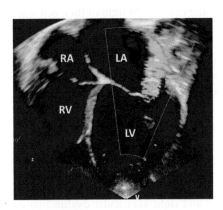

FIGURE 2

DCM seen from the apical four-chamber view. Dilatation of the left ventricle causes the mitral valve annulus to stretch, resulting in incomplete coaptation of the leaflets and mitral regurgitation. *LA*, left atrium; *LV*, left ventricle; *RA*, right atrium; *RV*, right ventricle.

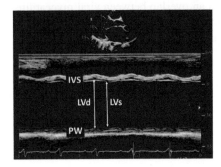

FIGURE 3

Parasternal long-axis M-mode demonstrating severe left ventricular (LV) dilatation and systolic dysfunction with minimal difference between the LV end-diastolic and end-systolic diameters. The resulting shortening fraction is barely measurable. *IVS*, interventricular septum interventricular septum; *LVd*, left ventricular end diastolic dimension; *LVs*, left ventricular end systolic dimension; *PW*, posterior wall.

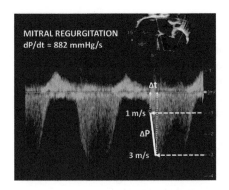

MITRAL REGURGITATION
dP/dt = 882 mmHg/s

1 m/s

ΔP

3 m/s

Δt

FIGURE 4

Continuous-wave Doppler of the mitral valve from the apical four-chamber view. The waveform of the regurgitant jet can be used to calculate **dP/dt**, a parameter reflecting the (early) left ventricular (LV) systolic function. According to the simplified Bernoulli equation, an increase in the flow velocity of the regurgitant jet from 1 to 3 m/s corresponds to an increase in systolic LV pressure of 32 mmHg. $[\Delta P = 4\ (3^2\,m/s - 1^2\,m/s) = 32\ mmHg]$. dP/dt is the ratio between this arbitrary selected pressure difference and the time it takes to reach it. Values >1200 mmHg/s are normal. In this example, dP/dt is 882 mmHg/s, which is consistent with LV systolic dysfunction. This parameter is however derived from velocity (dV/dt) hence dependent on loading conditions.

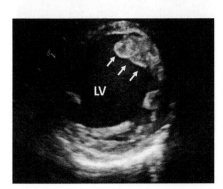

LV

FIGURE 5

Parasternal short axis view demonstrating a mural thrombus (*arrows*) in a child with DCM and severely decreased systolic function of the left ventricle (LV).

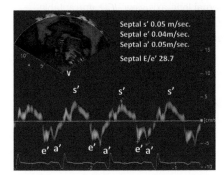

Septal s' 0.05 m/sec.
Septal e' 0.04m/sec.
Septal a' 0.05m/sec.

Septal E/e' 28.7

v

s'   s'   s'

e' a'   e' a'   e' a'

FIGURE 6

Pulsed-wave tissue Doppler at the level of the septal mitral valve annulus showing the velocity over time (see Chapter 1, Figure 49 for more details). In this patient with DCM, the s' wave amplitude is decreased to 0.05 m/s (normal value >0.08 m/s), which is consistent with systolic dysfunction. In addition, there is an increased E/e' ratio of 28.7 reflecting severe diastolic dysfunction. (pulsed-wave Doppler of transmitral flow and the measurement of E-wave amplitude are not shown).

Hypertrophic cardiomyopathy

The key feature of hypertrophic cardiomyopathy (HCM) is the presence of left ventricular hypertrophy that is not secondary to valvar disease, hypertension, or other cardiac diseases, which would be sufficient to result in a similar degree of hypertrophy. From a pathological point of view, this entity is characterized by an abnormal arrangement of heart muscle cells and fibrosis. It is commonly caused by mutations in genes coding for sarcomeric proteins.

The distribution of myocardial hypertrophy forms the essence of various subsets of HCM. Myocardial thickness should be measured in diastole from the parasternal short- or long-axis views. Measurements exceeding two standard deviations (indexed to body surface area) are considered abnormal. The morphology of the interventricular septum may form a substrate for dynamic left ventricular outflow tract obstruction due to systolic anterior motion of the anterior mitral valve leaflet.

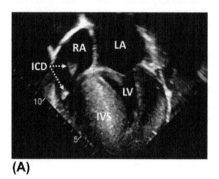 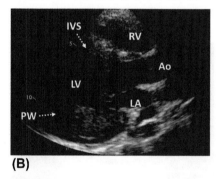

(A) **(B)**

FIGURE 7

(A) Apical four-chamber view. HCM with symmetrical hypertrophy of left ventricular (LV) myocardium. There is a reduction in the LV cavity size due to hypertrophy. Note the presence of an implantable cardioverter-defibrillator (ICD) lead crossing the tricuspid valve. (B) Same heart visualized from the parasternal long-axis view. *ICD*, implantable cardioverter defibrillator; *IVS*, interventricular septum; *LA*, left atrium; *LV*, left ventricle; *PW*, posterior wall; *RA*, right atrium; *RV*, right ventricle.

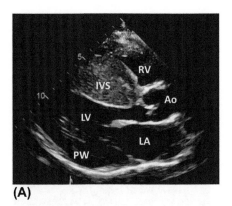 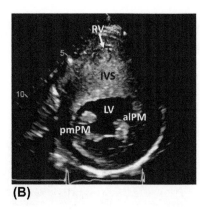

(A) **(B)**

FIGURE 8

(A) HCM seen from the parasternal long-axis view. There is asymmetric septal hypertrophy with normal left ventricular posterior wall thickness. (B) Same heart seen from the parasternal short-axis view. Note the extreme septal hypertrophy. *alPM*, antero-lateral papillary muscle; *Ao*, aorta; *IVS*, interventricular septum; *LA*, left atrium; *LV*, left ventricle; *RV*, right ventricle; *pmPM*, postero-medial papillary muscle; *PW*, posterior wall.

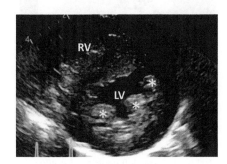

FIGURE 9

In HCM, papillary muscles are often malformed, abnormally rotated, or increased in number. Parasternal short-axis view showing three papillary muscles (*asterisks*) in the left ventricle. *LV*, left ventricle; *RV*, right ventricle.

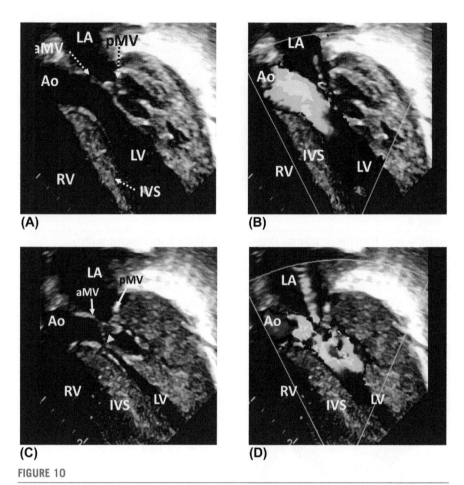

FIGURE 10

Child with HCM. Apical five-chamber view demonstrating dynamic left ventricular outflow tract (LVOT) obstruction due to systolic anterior motion (SAM) of the anterior mitral valve leaflet. (A) The hypertrophied interventricular septum bulges into LVOT. (B) As a result, there is mildly turbulent flow across the LVOT at the beginning of the systole. Note the mild degree of mitral regurgitation. (C) With the progression of systole, there is the displacement of the distal portion of the anterior mitral valve leaflet against the interventricular septum (*yellow arrowhead*). The anterior motion of the leaflet is due to the Venturi effect. (D) This increases the obstruction across the LVOT and aggravates the degree of mitral regurgitation. *aMV*, anterior leaflet of the mitral valve; *Ao*, aorta; *IVS*, interventricular septum; *LA*, left atrium; *LV*, left ventricle; *pMV*, posterior leaflet of the mitral valve; *RA*, right atrium.

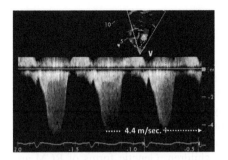

FIGURE 11

Continuous-wave Doppler of the left ventricular outflow tract from the apical five-chamber view. There is severe left ventricular outflow tract obstruction caused by the systolic anterior motion of the anterior mitral valve leaflet. In midsystole, the obstruction reaches its peak.

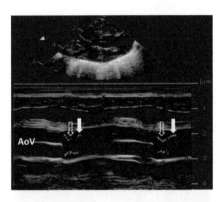

FIGURE 12

Parasternal long axis M-mode demonstrating mid-systolic closure of the aortic valve (AoV) in a patient with severe HCM. This premature aortic valve closure (*hollow arrow*) occurs due to severe left ventricular outflow tract obstruction caused by the systolic anterior motion of the anterior mitral valve leaflet. *White arrow* indicates the reopening of the valve toward the end of the systole when the level of dynamic obstruction decreases.

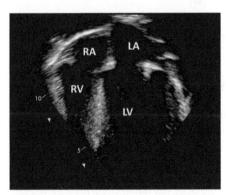

(A)

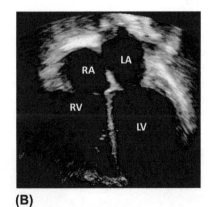

(B)

FIGURE 13

(A) Apical four-chamber view in a child with a severe form of HCM. (B) Progression of the disease in the same patient. The appearance of the left ventricle is similar to that of dilated cardiomyopathy, with marked left ventricular dilatation and dysfunction. *LA*, left atrium; *LV*, left ventricle; *RA*, right atrium; *RV*, right ventricle.

Restrictive cardiomyopathy

Restrictive cardiomyopathy (RCM) is a rare condition affecting one or both ventricles. It is characterized by an increased myocardial stiffness resulting in impaired ventricular filling and atrial dilatation. Unlike the diastolic function, the systolic function is often preserved. Ventricular volumes are usually reduced but may be normal. The thickness of the ventricular myocardium is not affected. In children, most cases of RCM are idiopathic, but can sometimes occur in patients with previous anthracycline therapy. In contrast to the adult population, cardiac amyloidosis, sarcoidosis, or hemochromatosis are rare in children. Genetic forms of RCM are very rare.

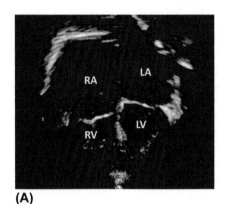
(A)

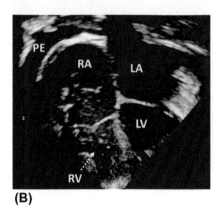
(B)

FIGURE 14

(A) Apical four-chamber view in a child with RCM. Note the small appearance of both ventricles. As a result of reduced compliance, there is severe biatrial enlargement. (B) Progression to end-stage disease in the same patient who in addition to diastolic dysfunction developed biventricular systolic dysfunction. There is spontaneous echo contrast in the right-sided chambers and new appearance of a pericardial effusion. *LA*, left atrium; *LV*, left ventricle; *PE*, pericardial effusion; *RA*, right atrium; *RV*, right ventricle.

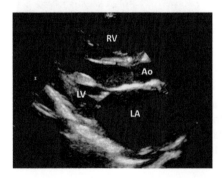

FIGURE 15

RCM seen from the parasternal long-axis view. Note the discrepancy between the severely enlarged left atrium and the small left ventricular cavity. *Ao*, aorta; *LA*, left atrium; *LV*, left ventricle; *RV*, right ventricle.

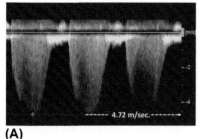 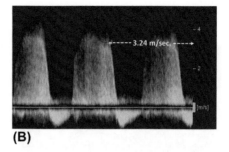

(A) **(B)**

FIGURE 16

Echocardiographic screening for pulmonary hypertension plays a key role in patients with RCM. A significant elevation of pulmonary vascular resistance may contraindicate cardiac transplantation. (A) Continuous-wave Doppler of the tricuspid valve demonstrating a high-velocity tricuspid regurgitation jet (peak velocity 4.72 m/s) consistent with an increase in the systolic pulmonary artery (PA) pressure. (B) High end-diastolic pulmonary regurgitation velocity (3.24 m/s) suggestive of a raised diastolic PA pressure. See Chapter 1, Figs. 45, 46 for further details on the calculation of PA pressures.

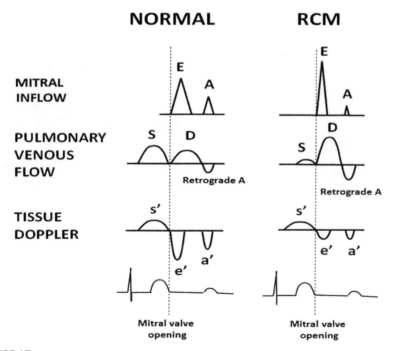

FIGURE 17

Restrictive filling pattern is demonstrated by changes in pulsed wave (PW) Doppler of the mitral inflow (E wave = early passive filling, A wave = late active filling); changes in PW Doppler of the **pulmonary and hepatic venous flow** (S wave = systolic flow, D wave = diastolic flow, A wave = retrograde flow during atrial contraction); and changes in PW tissue Doppler (s' wave = systolic movement of the mitral annulus, e' wave = early diastolic movement of the mitral annulus, a' wave = movement of the mitral annulus due to the atrial contraction).

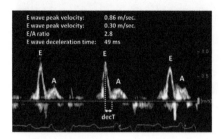

FIGURE 18

Pulsed wave (PW) Doppler of mitral inflow from the apical four-chamber view. In a normal heart, ventricular filling occurs predominantly during the early passive phase of diastole rather than the late active phase. The E wave is, therefore, taller than the A wave. However, in RCM high end-diastolic ventricular pressure caused by increased myocardial stiffness results in rapid equalization of ventricular and atrial diastolic pressure and marked shortening of the passive filling phase. The atrial contraction plays a minimal role in the ventricular filling because the dilated atrium is unable to generate sufficient pressure to further fill the stiff ventricle. Thus, the E wave becomes very tall compared to the A wave and the E/A ratio increases (E/A >2). The time required for the early diastolic flow (E wave) to decrease from peak to zero, called the deceleration time (decT), is substantially reduced (<150 ms). This figure shows mitral inflow PW Doppler in a child with RCM. In this example, the E/A ratio is 2.8 and the decT is 49 ms.

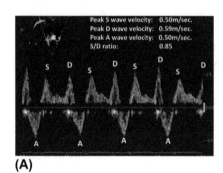
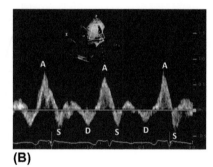

(A) **(B)**

FIGURE 19

(A) Pulsed-wave Doppler of the right lower pulmonary vein from the apical four-chamber view. Under normal circumstances, the pulmonary venous flow is more prominent in systole than in diastole. Thus, the S wave is taller than the D wave. However, in RCM, the elevated left atrial pressure reduces the systolic flow while the diastolic flow becomes more pronounced. As a result, the S wave/D wave ratio decreases (below 1.0). Rather than contributing to the ventricular filling, the atrial contraction leads to an increase in the retrograde flow (A wave). (B) The hepatic venous flow is analogous to the pulmonary venous flow. Pulsed-wave Doppler of the hepatic vein from the subcostal approach. Note the very prominent retrograde A wave consistent with a restrictive filling pattern.

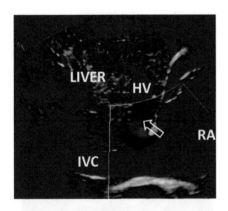

FIGURE 20

Subcostal view showing retrograde hepatic venous flow (*arrow*) during atrial systole in a child with RCM. *HV*, hepatic vein; *IVC*, inferior vena cava; *RA*, right atrium.

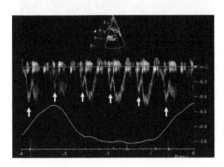

FIGURE 21

Pulsed-wave Doppler of the pulmonary artery in a child with restrictive filling of the right ventricle. The *white arrows* represent an antegrade end-diastolic flow in the pulmonary artery caused by right atrial contraction. The amplitude of the atrial contraction detected in the pulmonary artery varies with respiration (light green line, upslope = inspiration, downslope = expiration). This feature is consistent with significant right ventricular diastolic dysfunction. However, in patients who have restriction not only of the right but also of the left ventricle, this sign may not be present due to high left atrial pressure leading to an elevation in the pulmonary artery pressure.

Courtesy of Professor Jan Marek.

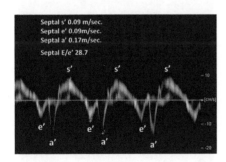

FIGURE 22

Pulsed-wave tissue Doppler at the level of the lateral mitral valve annulus demonstrating an increased E/e' ratio of 28.7, consistent with severe diastolic dysfunction in this child with RCM. (Pulsed-wave Doppler of the transmitral flow and measurement of the E wave amplitude are not shown). The s' wave velocity is 0.09 m/s, indicating preserved systolic function.

Noncompaction cardiomyopathy

Left ventricular noncompaction cardiomyopathy is characterized by the presence of prominent ventricular trabeculae and recesses. The myocardium is usually thickened, with the compacted (epicardial) layer being much thinner than the noncompacted (endocardial) layer. Some patients develop systolic dysfunction with disease progression.

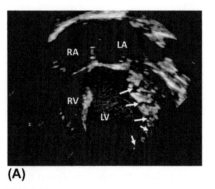
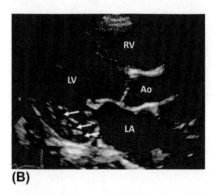

(A)   (B)

FIGURE 23

(A) Apical four-chamber view of left ventricular noncompaction cardiomyopathy. The myocardium has a spongy appearance, with marked trabeculations and deep recesses (*arrows*). The left ventricle is severely dilated and dysfunctional. (B) Same heart seen from the parasternal long-axis view. *LA*, left atrium; *LV*, left ventricle; *RA*, right atrium; *RV*, right ventricle; Ao aorta.

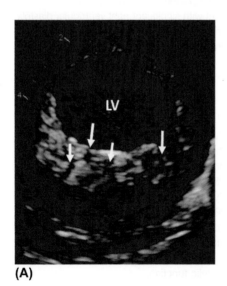
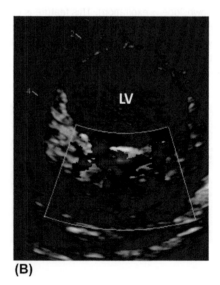

(A)   (B)

FIGURE 24

(A) Noncompaction cardiomyopathy demonstrated from the parasternal short-axis view. The *arrows* indicate deep recesses in the left ventricular (LV) myocardium. The thickness of the compacted layer is modest compared to the noncompacted layer. (B) Blood flow into the recesses as shown on color flow mapping.

Kawasaki disease

23

Kawasaki disease is one of the most frequent childhood vasculitides affecting medium-sized muscular arteries and in particular coronary arteries. The etiology of this condition remains unknown. However, the clinical picture and the epidemiology suggest an infectious cause with no pathogen identified so far. The hallmark of Kawasaki disease is high fever with poor response to antipyretics or antibiotics. The diagnosis relies on the recognition of the clinical features, laboratory investigations, and echocardiography or other imaging modalities.

Detectable changes to the coronary arteries by echocardiography usually appear 2–3 weeks after the onset of fever, rarely developing within the first 10 days or after the first 6 weeks of the disease. Coronary artery abnormalities seen in Kawasaki disease include coronary ectasia and saccular or fusiform aneurysms. Usually, proximal coronary arteries are affected, whereas distal coronary artery involvement without proximal changes is uncommon. The size and the number of the lesions is variable and can range from small to giant aneurysms (>8 mm), affecting one or multiple segments.

Acute coronary artery thrombosis is a rare but life-threatening complication of the disease. Unlike occlusive thrombosis, nonocclusive laminar thrombosis is relatively common and develops often in patients with giant aneurysms many years after the onset of the disease.

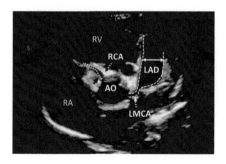

FIGURE 1

Parasternal short-axis view demonstrating a giant fusiform aneurysm of the left anterior descending coronary artery (LAD) (*double arrow, dashed lines*). There is also mild dilatation (*black arrow*) of the proximal right coronary artery (RCA) (*dotted lines*). The left main coronary artery (LMCA) is of normal caliber. *Ao*, aorta; *RA*, right atrium; *RV*, right ventricle.

Atlas of Pediatric Echocardiography. https://doi.org/10.1016/B978-0-323-75981-6.00033-9

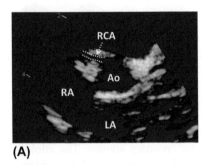 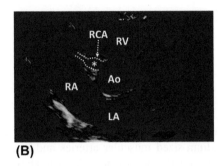

(A) **(B)**

FIGURE 2

Parasternal short-axis view showing the development of an aneurysm in the proximal right coronary artery (RCA). (A) Initial echocardiogram demonstrating the normal appearance of the right coronary artery (*dotted lines*). (B) Same patient a week later. *Asterisk* indicates a newly developed proximal RCA aneurysm. *Ao*, aorta; *LA*, left aorta; *RA*, right atrium; *RV*, right ventricle.

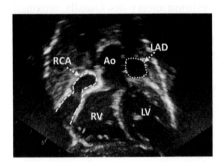

FIGURE 3

Subcostal long-axis view demonstrating giant fusiform aneurysms (*dashed lines*) of the right coronary artery (RCA) and the left anterior descending coronary artery (LAD). The latter is seen en face. Note the absence of mural thrombi. *Ao*, aorta; *LV*, left ventricle; *RV*, right ventricle.

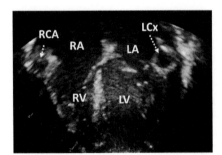

FIGURE 4

Zoomed apical four-chamber view showing aneurysms of the right coronary artery (RCA) and the left circumflex coronary artery (LCx). *LA*, left atrium; *LV*, left ventricle; *RA*, right atrium; *RV*, right ventricle.

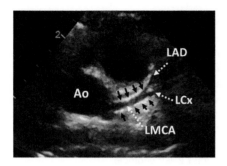

FIGURE 5

Parasternal short-axis view demonstrating perivascular echo brightness (*black arrows*) of the left main coronary artery (LMCA). Perivascular echo brightness was previously considered as a marker of inflammation. However, current guidelines do not support its use in therapeutic decision making as it is a subjective and poorly reproducible parameter. *Ao*, aorta; *LAD*, left anterior descending coronary artery; *LCx*, left circumflex coronary artery.

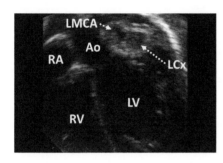

FIGURE 6

Acute left coronary artery thrombosis visualized from the apical five-chamber view. There is a complex giant aneurysm involving the bifurcation of the left coronary artery. The circumflex branch of the left coronary artery (LCx) is completely filled with an occlusive thrombus. There is a nonocclusive thrombus in the left main coronary artery (LMCA). *Ao*, aorta; *LV*, left ventricle; *RA*, right atrium; *RV*, right ventricle.

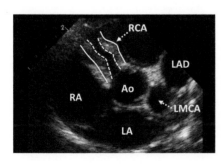

FIGURE 7

Parasternal short-axis view illustrating a nonocclusive laminar thrombus in a giant fusiform aneurysm of the right coronary artery (RCA). The solid lines represent the walls of the aneurysmal coronary artery. The dashed lines correspond to the effective lumen of the right coronary artery. The thrombus is located between the dashed and the solid lines. There is also a giant aneurysm of the left main (LMCA) and left anterior descending coronary artery (LAD). *Ao*, aorta, *LA*, left atrium, *RA*, right atrium.

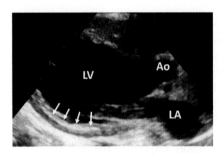

FIGURE 8

Parasternal long-axis view in a patient who suffered from an acute myocardial infarction following an episode of Kawasaki disease. Despite urgent surgical revascularization, the child developed severe hypokinesia of the left ventricular posterior wall. Note hyperechogenicity of the affected segments. *Ao*, aorta; *LA*, left atrium; *LV*, left ventricle.

Rheumatic fever

24

Acute rheumatic fever is an autoimmune disease triggered by a group A Streptococcal pharyngitis. It usually leads to multisystem involvement starting a few weeks after the initial Streptococcal infection. The most worrisome complication of acute rheumatic fever is **acute rheumatic carditis**, which develops in approximately half of the patients. It mainly affects the endocardium of the mitral valve and less frequently the aortic valve. Pericardial and myocardial involvement may also be present. Apart from aortic regurgitation, these changes usually resolve.

The term **rheumatic heart disease** refers to the development of permanent and irreversible cardiac damage that occurs years after one severe or multiple episodes of acute rheumatic fever. It is an important cause of cardiac morbidity and mortality in children in developing countries. Rheumatic heart disease almost exclusively affects the mitral and the aortic valves. Tricuspid valve pathology is rare and the pulmonary valve is typically spared.

The disease process is characterized by scarring of the heart valves and their subvalvar apparatus, leading to stenosis and regurgitation. The key echocardiographic features include valvar thickening, chordal fusion and shortening, commissural fusion, and calcifications.

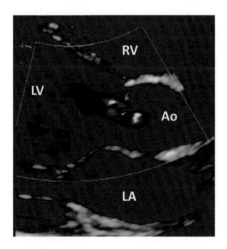

FIGURE 1

Zoomed parasternal long-axis view in a child with subclinical acute rheumatic carditis. There is mild aortic and trivial mitral regurgitation as visualized on color flow Doppler. *Ao*, aorta; *LA*, left atrium; *LV*, left ventricle; *RV*, right ventricle.

Atlas of Pediatric Echocardiography. https://doi.org/10.1016/B978-0-323-75981-6.00017-0

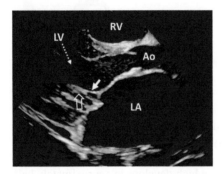

FIGURE 2

Zoomed parasternal long-axis view in a patient with severe mixed mitral valve disease in the context of chronic rheumatic heart disease. The chordae tendineae supporting the mitral valve are thickened, shortened (*white arrow*), and fused (*hollow arrow*), resulting in reduced motion of the leaflets. The left atrium is dilated due to significant mitral regurgitation. *Ao*, aorta; *LA*, left atrium; *LV*, left ventricle; *RV*, right ventricle.

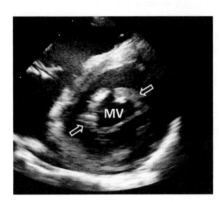

FIGURE 3

Parasternal short-axis view at the level of the mitral valve (MV) orifice in a patient with rheumatic heart disease and severe mitral stenosis. The valve is thickened and there is commissural fusion (*hollow arrows*) restricting the opening of the leaflets.

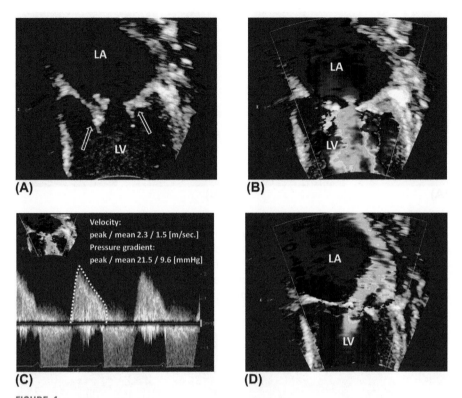

(A)   **(B)**

(C)   **(D)**

Velocity:
peak / mean 2.3 / 1.5 [m/sec.]
Pressure gradient:
peak / mean 21.5 / 9.6 [mmHg]

FIGURE 4

Severe mixed mitral valve disease in a child with rheumatic heart disease. (A) Zoomed apical four-chamber view showing thickened, scarred, and calcified mitral valve leaflets (*hollow arrows*). (B) The leaflets are restricted in motion which results in turbulent flow across the valve, as evidenced on color flow mapping. (C) Continuous-wave Doppler of the mitral valve showing a significantly increased transvalvar gradient of 21.5/9.6 mmHg (peak/mean gradient). (D) Severe mitral regurgitation because of damage to the valve and the subvalvar apparatus. As a consequence, there is a significant left atrial dilatation. *LA*, left atrium; *LV*, left ventricle.

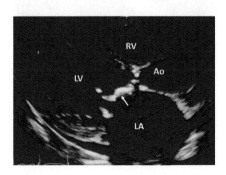

FIGURE 5

Mitral valve stenosis due to rheumatic heart disease. Parasternal long-axis view demonstrating thickening of the leaflets. The orifice of the valve is funnel-shaped (*doming*). There is a "dog leg" appearance of the anterior leaflet (*arrow*). Note the significant thickening and scarring of the aortic valve. *LA*, left atrium; *LV*, left ventricle; *RV*, right.

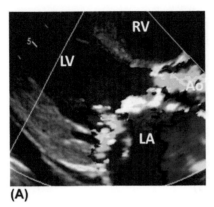 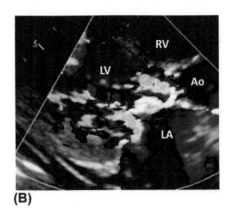

(A) (B)

FIGURE 6

Zoomed parasternal long-axis view in a child with mixed mitral and aortic valve disease. (A) In systole, there is turbulent flow across the aortic valve and significant posteriorly directed mitral regurgitation. This results in left ventricular hypertrophy and left atrial dilatation. (B) In diastole, there is turbulent flow across the mitral valve and significant aortic regurgitation. *Ao*, aorta; *LA*, left atrium; *LV*, left ventricle; *RV*, right ventricle.

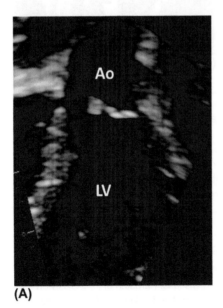 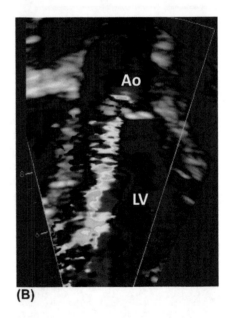

(A) (B)

FIGURE 7

Zoomed parasternal five-chamber view showing the aortic valve in a patient with rheumatic heart disease. (A) The valve is thickened and has an irregular appearance. (B) Note the severe aortic regurgitation as demonstrated on color flow mapping. *Ao*, aorta, *LV*, left ventricle.

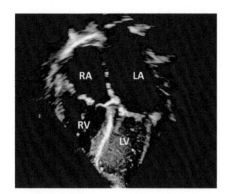

FIGURE 8

Apical four-chamber view in a child with rheumatic heart disease and severe involvement of the mitral and tricuspid valves. Both valves appear thickened and scarred. The left atrium is severely dilated due to mitral regurgitation. *LA*, left atrium; *LV*, left ventricle; *RA*, right atrium; *RV*, right ventricle.

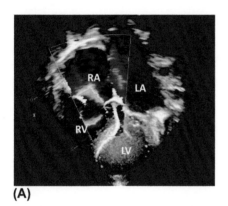

(A)

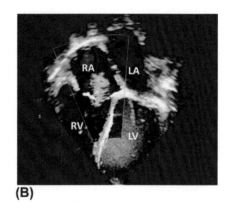

(B)

FIGURE 9

(A) Apical four-chamber view in a child with rheumatic heart disease and severe mixed tricuspid valve disease. Color flow Doppler demonstrating turbulent flow across the valve in diastole. (B) In systole, there is significant tricuspid regurgitation. *LA*, left atrium; *LV*, left ventricle; *RA*, right atrium; *RV*, right ventricle.

Infective endocarditis (IE)

25

The term infective endocarditis (IE) refers to an infection of the endocardial surface of the heart, affecting the cardiac valves, mural endocardium, and septal defects. In most cases, the infection is caused by bacteria, but a fungal etiology is also possible. It is a life-threatening condition that despite antibiotic treatment, can rapidly develop into a hemodynamic collapse. IE often leads to damage of the heart valves and their subvalvar apparatus, resulting in uncontrollable regurgitation.

Risk factors for infective endocarditis include structural heart disease (repaired or unrepaired) and the presence of foreign material such as prosthetic valves, conduits, homografts, pacemaker leads, interventional devices, or central venous lines. IE is often induced by transient bacteremia caused, for example, by dental procedures or intravenous drug abuse.

The echocardiographic diagnosis is based on the detection of vegetations or abscesses. In patients with prosthetic valves, IE may manifest as valvar dehiscence or malfunction. In many cases, there are no compelling echocardiographic features despite repeatedly positive blood cultures in at-risk patients.

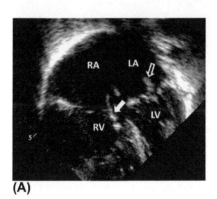 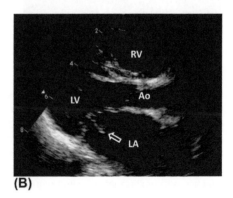

(A) **(B)**

FIGURE 1

(A) Apical four-chamber view in a patient with previous cardiac surgery for complete atrio-ventricular septal defect. There is a vegetation on the left atrio-ventricular valve (*hollow arrow*). The *solid white arrow* indicates the pericardial patch closing the atrial and ventricular component. (B) Same vegetation (*hollow arrow*) seen from the parasternal long-axis view. *Ao*, aorta; *LA*, left atrium; *LV*, left ventricle; *RA*, right atrium; *RV*, right ventricle.

Atlas of Pediatric Echocardiography. https://doi.org/10.1016/B978-0-323-75981-6.00018-2

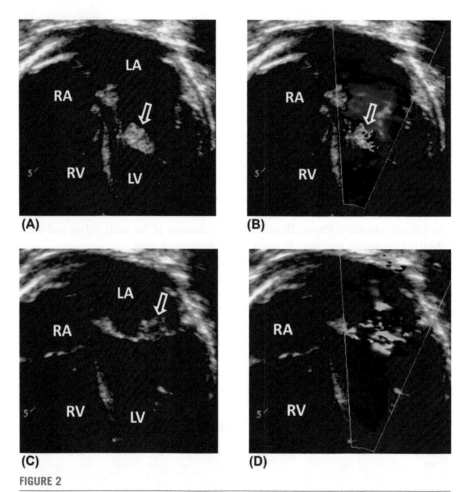

FIGURE 2

(A) Zoomed apical four-chamber view showing a large flailing vegetation (*hollow arrow*) on the anterior leaflet of the mitral valve in a previously fit and well child with a recent history of tonsillitis. The vegetation is attached to the leaflet by a narrow base. (B) Color flow Doppler showing no evidence of obstruction to mitral inflow caused by the vegetation. (C) Systolic frame illustrating the close relationship of the vegetation (*hollow arrow*) to the zone of coaptation. (D) There is an extensive area of leaflet perforation caused by the infection with multiple jets of mitral regurgitation. *LA*, left atrium; *LV*, left ventricle; *RA*, right atrium; *RV*, right ventricle.

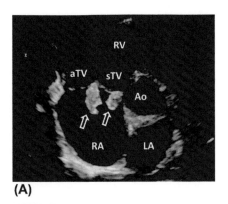 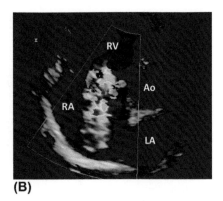

(A) **(B)**

FIGURE 3

(A) Parasternal short-axis view illustrating large vegetations on the anterior and septal leaflets of the tricuspid valve (*hollow arrows*) in a patient with no previous history of cardiac surgery. (B) Note the erosion of the leaflets caused by the disease, leading to severe tricuspid regurgitation as demonstrated on color flow Doppler. *Ao*, aorta; *aTV*, antero-superior tricuspid valve leaflet; *LA*, left atrium; *RA*, right atrium; *RV*, right ventricle; *sTV*, septal tricuspid valve leaflet.

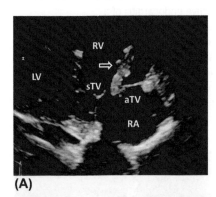 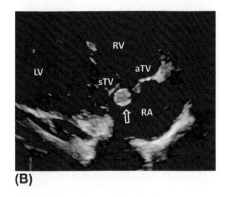

(A) **(B)**

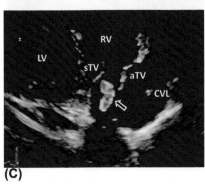

(C)

FIGURE 4

(A) Parasternal long-axis view of the tricuspid valve showing a large flailing vegetation on the antero-superior tricuspid valve leaflet (*hollow arrow*). (B and C) Due to ruptured chordal attachments, there is an extensive systolic prolapse of the anterior leaflet, along with the vegetation (*hollow arrow*), into the right atrium. *Ao*, aorta; *aTV*, antero-superior tricuspid valve leaflet; *LV*, left ventricle; *RA*, right atrium; *RV*, right ventricle; *sTV*, septal tricuspid valve leaflet.

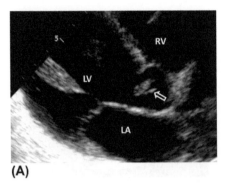
(A)

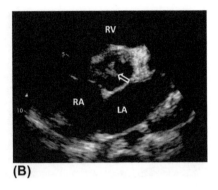
(B)

FIGURE 5

(A) Parasternal long-axis view demonstrating an aortic valve vegetation (*hollow arrow*) in a patient with Streptococcus pneumoniae endocarditis. (B) Same vegetation (*hollow arrow*) seen from the parasternal short-axis view. *LA*, left atrium; *LV*, left ventricle; *RA*, right atrium; *RV*, right ventricle.

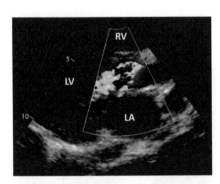

FIGURE 6

Parasternal long-axis view in a patient with infective endocarditis of a quadricommissural aortic valve in cardiogenic shock. Note the complete destruction of the leaflets resulting in severe aortic regurgitation, as evidenced on color flow Doppler. *LA*, left atrium; *LV*, left ventricle; *RV*, right ventricle.

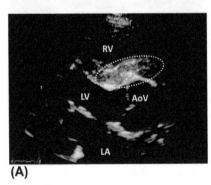
(A)

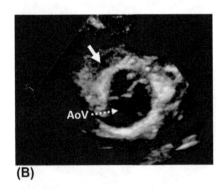
(B)

FIGURE 7

(A) Parasternal long-axis view demonstrating an abscess of the aortic root (*dotted oval*). (B) Same pathology seen from a zoomed parasternal short-axis view. Note the hypoechogenic center of the lesion (*arrow*) suggestive of abscess cavity formation. Surgical replacement of the aortic root was required in this child. *AoV*, aortic valve; *LA*, left atrium; *LV*, left ventricle; *RV*, right ventricle.

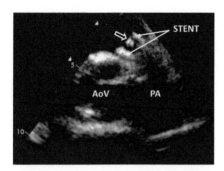

FIGURE 8

Infective endocarditis of a percutaneously implanted pulmonary valve with an in-stent vegetation (*hollow arrow*) seen from a zoomed parasternal short-axis view. This patient had multiple previous interventions for common arterial trunk. *AoV*, aortic valve; *PA*, pulmonary artery.

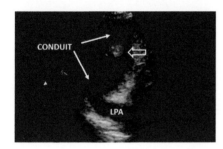

FIGURE 9

Focused parasternal short-axis view in a child with infective endocarditis of a conduit in the pulmonary position. There is a large vegetation (*hollow arrow*) attached to the wall of the conduit. This child had previous cardiac surgery for tetralogy of Fallot with pulmonary atresia. *LPA*, left pulmonary artery.

Pericardial disease

26

The pericardium is a double-layered fibroelastic sac that surrounds the heart and the roots of the great vessels. Under normal circumstances, the pericardial cavity is filled with a small amount of fluid that lubricates the heart and reduces friction against the surrounding structures.

An imbalance between the production and the absorption of pericardial fluid leads to the development of a pericardial effusion. In extreme cases, this can result in **cardiac tamponade** and subsequent circulatory collapse. **Acute pericarditis** is a common cause of pericardial effusion in the pediatric population, while **constrictive pericarditis** is rarely encountered in children nowadays.

Acute pericarditis and pericardial effusion

Acute pericarditis is an inflammation of the pericardium that usually results in excessive production of pericardial fluid. Most often this is caused by a viral or bacterial infection, but a noninfectious etiology including autoimmune disease, radiation, cancer, or trauma is also not uncommon. Furthermore, pericardial effusion may develop in severely malnourished children or following cardiac procedures.

In acute pericarditis, the pericardium is thickened and hyperechogenic. Echocardiography can also provide an estimate of the type of effusion. Serous effusions have an echo-free appearance, while hemorrhagic or purulent effusions are usually echo dense and echogenic. Fibrin deposits, strands, and septae may also be present.

Atlas of Pediatric Echocardiography. https://doi.org/10.1016/B978-0-323-75981-6.00001-7

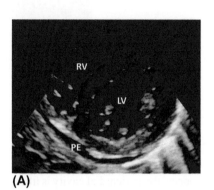 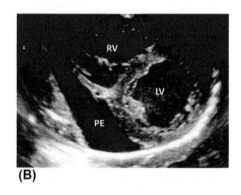

(A)   **(B)**

FIGURE 1

(A) Parasternal short-axis views demonstrating a small rim of pericardial effusion in a patient with myopericarditis. The pericardium has an echo bright appearance. (B) Moderate pericardial effusion in a child with systemic onset juvenile idiopathic arthritis. *LV*, left ventricle; *PE*, pericardial effusion; *RV*, right ventricle.

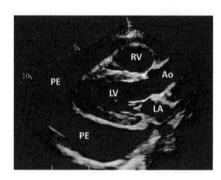

FIGURE 2

Parasternal long-axis view showing a "floating heart" in a patient with a systemic connective tissue disorder. In this case, the absence of clinical or echocardiographic signs of cardiac tamponade suggests a slow accumulation of the pericardial fluid. The chronic nature of the process allowed pericardial distension without significantly increasing the intrapericardial pressure. *Ao*, aorta; *LA*, left atrium; *LV*, left ventricle; *PE*, pericardial effusion; *RV*, right ventricle.

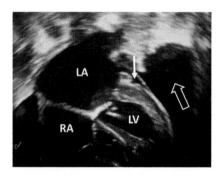

FIGURE 3

Subcostal four-chamber view demonstrating a large echo-free space (*hollow arrow*) that mimicks a significant pericardial effusion. However, this corresponds to a large left-sided pleural effusion. There is a small physiological amount of pericardial fluid seen in the left atrio-ventricular groove (*white arrow*) with no separation between the inner and outer layer of pericardium. *LA*, left atrium; *LV*, left ventricle; *RA*, right atrium.

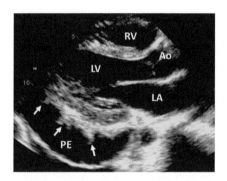

FIGURE 4

Large pericardial effusion in an immunocompromised child visualized from the parasternal long-axis view. Note the presence of hyperechogenic fibrin deposits and strands (*arrows*) indicating possible bacterial etiology. *Ao*, aorta; *LA*, left atrium, *LV*, left ventricle; *PE*, pericardial effusion; *RV*, right ventricle.

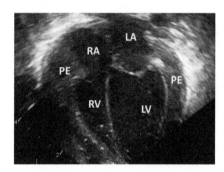

FIGURE 5

Purulent pericardial effusion seen from the apical four-chamber view. Note the echo-dense layer between the parietal and visceral pericardium, surrounding all the heart chambers. Pneumococcal etiology was subsequently confirmed. *LA*, left atrium; *LV*, left ventricle; *PE*, pericardial effusion; *RA*, right atrium; *RV*, right ventricle.

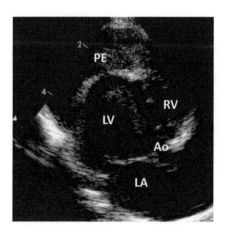

FIGURE 6

Modified parasternal long-axis view demonstrating a large echo-dense pericardial effusion in a patient with tuberculosis. The effusion is mainly located in front of the apex of the heart. *LA*, left atrium; *LV*, left ventricle; *PE*, pericardial effusion; *RA*, right atrium; *RV*, right ventricle.

Cardiac tamponade

Cardiac tamponade is a life-threatening condition characterized by compression of the heart by pericardial fluid. Rapid accumulation of even a small amount of fluid in the pericardial cavity can sometimes lead to a significant increase in the intrapericardial pressure. This is due to a limited distensibility of the pericardium. The right atrium and ventricle are the first cardiac chambers to collapse because of their low pressures in late and early diastole, respectively. On the other hand, if the accumulation of the pericardial fluid is slow enough to allow pericardial remodeling and distension, even a large volume of fluid may have a minimal hemodynamic impact. Echocardiographic features of diastolic dysfunction and impaired diastolic filling are discussed in more detail in Chapter 22 on cardiomyopathies (section on restrictive cardiomyopathy).

Under normal circumstances, the inspiratory drop in intrathoracic pressure causes the systemic venous return to increase, resulting in better filling of the right atrium and ventricle. Due to the fixed volume of the pericardial cavity, the filling of the left heart as well as the left ventricular stroke volume is reduced. The opposite is true for expiration. This phenomenon is called ventricular interdependence (Figure 7).

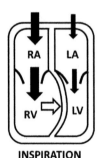 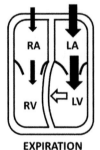

INSPIRATION   **EXPIRATION**

FIGURE 7

Ventricular interdependance.

In cardiac tamponade, the above described respiratory variations are exaggerated. The filling of the right heart is impaired due to its collapse and becomes heavily dependent on inspiration driving the systemic venous return. In tamponade, the peak early tricuspid inflow velocity (E wave) drops by >40% in expiration compared to inspiration. Similarly, the peak early mitral inflow velocity drops by >25% in inspiration compared to expiration. Analogously, this applies to the left ventricular outflow and abdominal aortic flow velocities, which can be used to diagnose paradoxical pulse in tamponade.

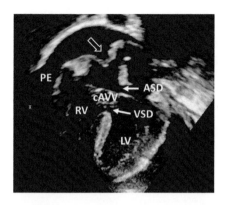

FIGURE 8

Apical four-chamber view in a child with complete atrio-ventricular septal defect and large pericardial effusion causing cardiac tamponade. There is right atrial collapse (*hollow arrow*) that becomes more pronounced on expiration when the systemic venous return is reduced. *ASD*, atrial septal defect; *cAVV*, common atrio-ventricular valve; *LV*, left ventricle; *PE*, pericardial effusion; *RV*, right ventricle; *VSD*, ventricular septal defect.

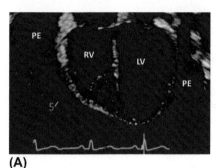

(A)

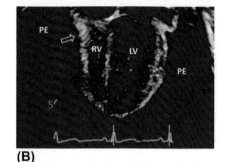

(B)

FIGURE 9

(A) Zoomed apical four-chamber view demonstrating an extremely large pericardial effusion ("floating heart"). In systole, the right ventricular pressure exceeds the intrapericardial pressure, hence, the right ventricle has a normal shape. (B) Early diastolic frame showing right ventricular free wall collapse (*hollow arrow*) due to the increased intrapericardial pressure. The extent and the duration of the collapse reflect the severity of tamponade. *LV*, left ventricle; *PE*, pericardial effusion; *RV*, right ventricle.

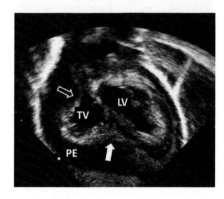

FIGURE 10

Subcostal four-chamber view showing right atrial (*hollow arrow*) and right ventricular (*white arrow*) collapse in a child with cardiac tamponade. *LV*, left ventricle; *PE*, pericardial effusion; *TV*, tricuspid valve.

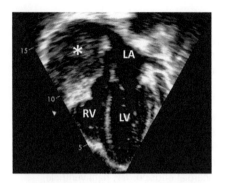

FIGURE 11

Postoperative hemopericardium with a large collection (asterisk) around the right atrium, and to some extent the ventricle, causing collapse. *LA*, left atrium; *LV*, left ventricle; *RA*, right atrium.

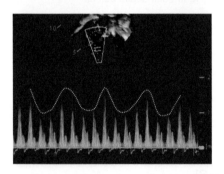

FIGURE 12

Pulsed-wave Doppler of the tricuspid inflow from the apical four-chamber view in a child with cardiac tamponade. In this trace, the E and A waves are fused. Note the exaggerated respiratory variation (*dotted line*) in the peak E wave velocity. The E wave is tallest in inspiration when the systemic venous return is highest and, by analogy, is smallest in expiration. In cardiac tamponade, the difference between the amplitude of the E wave in inspiration compared to expiration exceeds 40%, as in this example.

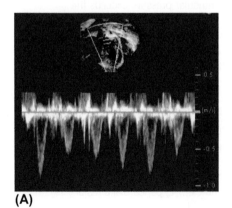

(A) **(B)**

FIGURE 13

(A) Paradoxical pulse in cardiac tamponade demonstrated by pulsed-wave Doppler of the left ventricular outflow tract from the apical five-chamber view. Note the changes in the amplitudes of the pulse waves with respiration. (B) Similar tracing obtained by pulsed-wave Doppler of the abdominal aorta from the subcostal approach. In both examples, the difference between the highest (expiratory) and the lowest (inspiratory) flow velocity exceeds 25%.

Constrictive pericarditis

Constrictive pericarditis is a rare chronic condition characterized by abnormal fibrous scarring of the pericardium that becomes thickened or even calcified. Any type of pericardial disease can lead to constrictive pericarditis, but most commonly it develops after bacterial pericarditis. Echocardiography plays a key role in making the distinction between constrictive pericarditis and restrictive cardiomyopathy, as they often show similar clinical and hemodynamic features. Unlike restrictive cardiomyopathy, constrictive pericarditis can often be treated surgically.

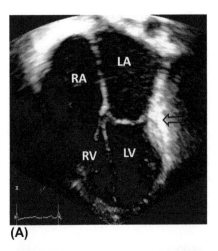

(A)

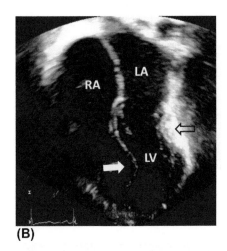

(B)

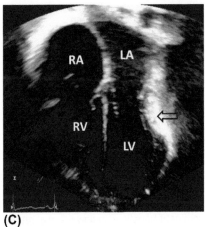

(C)

FIGURE 14

Apical four-chamber view showing abnormal septal motion in a patient with constrictive pericarditis. Note the thickened and calcified pericardium (*hollow arrow*). (A) Increased systemic venous return during inspiration causes premature opening of the tricuspid valve. (B) Due to a fixed pericardial volume in constrictive pericarditis, the ventricular interdependence is exaggerated. An increase in right ventricular filling during inspiration leads to a reduction in the left ventricular preload. This produces a diastolic septal bounce (*white arrow*).

(C) The interventricular septum moves to the normal midline position in late diastole. *LA,* left atrium; *LV,* left ventricle; *RA,* right atrium; *RV,* right ventricle.

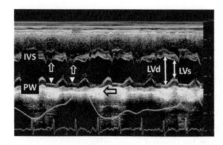

FIGURE 15

Parasternal short-axis M-mode demonstrating exaggerated ventricular interdependence in a child with constrictive pericarditis. *White hollow arrows* indicate the inspiratory septal bounce associated with flattening of the left ventricular posterior wall (arrow heads). Respiration is represented by the green line (upslope = inspiration, downslope = expiration). Note the thickening and calcification of the pericardium (*black hollow arrow*). IVS, interventricular septum; LV, left ventricular end-diastolic diameter; LV, ventricular end-systolic diameter; PW, posterior wall.

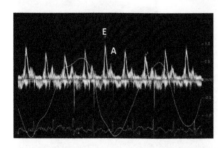

FIGURE 16

Pulsed-wave Doppler of mitral inflow from the apical four-chamber view in a patient with constrictive pericarditis. This example shows exaggerated ventricular interdependence with >25% drop in the peak E wave velocity during inspiration compared to expiration. This change is most evident in the first two beats of inspiration. Respiration is represented by the green line (upslope = inspiration, downslope = expiration). E wave = early passive filling, A wave = late active filling.

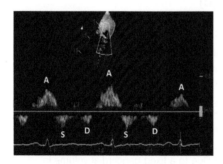

FIGURE 17

One of the differences between constrictive pericarditis and restrictive cardiomyopathy (RCM) is the flow pattern in the hepatic veins. In constrictive pericarditis, due to exaggerated interventricular dependence, the interventricular septum moves toward the right ventricle (RV) in expiration, thus reducing the RV filling capacity. As a result, the atrial contraction will lead to an increase in the hepatic vein flow reversal, that is, the amplitude of the A wave. Analogously, the amplitude of the A wave will decrease in inspiration. However, in RCM ventricular pressures are concordant, but the ventricular filling capacity is limited due to myocardial stiffness. During inspiration, when the RV preload is increased, atrial contraction will result in a more prominent hepatic vein flow reversal rather than an increase in ventricular filling. Unlike in constrictive pericarditis, where the A wave is tallest in expiration, in RCM, the A wave is tallest during inspiration. Figure 18 represents pulsed-wave Doppler of the hepatic veins from the subcostal view in a child with constrictive pericarditis. Note the respiratory variation of the A wave amplitude. (See Chapter 1, Figures 42, 43 for more details).

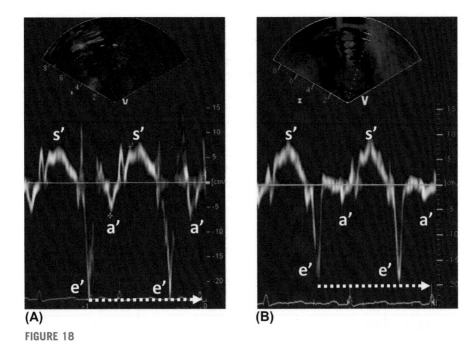

(A)   **(B)**

FIGURE 18

Pulsed-wave (PW) tissue Doppler at the level of the (A) septal and (B) lateral mitral valve annulus in a patient with constrictive pericarditis. Under normal circumstances, the early diastolic mitral annular velocity (e′ wave) measured from the lateral annulus is higher than the velocity from the septal annulus. The opposite is true in constrictive pericarditis, probably due to tethering of the lateral mitral annulus to the pericardium. This phenomenon is called "annulus reversus." (See Chapter 1, image 49 for more details on tissue Doppler imaging.)

Table 1 Echocardiographic features in constrictive pericarditis, cardiac tamponade, and restrictive cardiomyopathy.

	Cardiac tamponade	Constrictive pericarditis	Restrictive cardiomyopathy
Two dimensional imaging	- Pericardial effusion - Diastolic right atrial and right ventricular collapse	- Thickened (calcified) pericardium - Moderate atrial dilatation often present	- Usually severe atrial dilatation - Usually small ventricle(s)
Septal motion	Abnormal (inspiratory septal bounce)	Abnormal (inspiratory septal bounce)	Normal
Mitral inflow	↗ respiratory variation in peak E velocity by >25%	↗ respiratory variation in peak E velocity by >25% - E/A ratio >1.5 - decT (ms) <150 ms	No ↗ respiratory variation of peak E velocity - E/A ratio >1.5 - decT (ms) < 150 ms
Tricuspid inflow	↗ respiratory variation in peak E velocity by >40%	↗ respiratory variation in peak E velocity by >40%	No ↗ respiratory variation of peak E velocity
Mitral tissue Doppler: - Septal e' - Lateral e'	Varies	>8 cm/s Smaller than septal e'	<8 cm/s Taller than septal e'
Hepatic vein Doppler	Expiratory flow reversal	Expiratory flow reversal	Inspiratory flow reversal
IVC	Dilated No collapse	Dilated No collapse	Dilated No collapse

decT, *deceleration time*, IVC, *inferior vena cava.*
↗ *means increase.*

Cardiac tumors

27

In children, most cases of primary heart tumors are benign, while malignant lesions are rare. The most common tumors in childhood include cardiac **rhabdomyoma** and **fibroma**. Cardiac **myxoma** is rarely diagnosed in the pediatric population. Secondary metastatic malignancies are uncommon in children, but represent the largest group of cardiac tumors in adults. There is an association between certain types of tumors and some genetic syndromes, that is, rhabdomyomas typically occur in patients with tuberous sclerosis, while fibromas are often seen in children with Gorlin syndrome.

The clinical presentation depends on a number of factors such as the location and the type of lesion. Large tumors may cause obstruction to blood flow or, if invasive, may result in cardiac dysfunction, arrhythmia, or the accumulation of pericardial fluid. Some tumors may embolize to the systemic or pulmonary circulation. Cardiac surgery is the treatment of choice in the majority of patients.

Rhabdomyoma

Cardiac rhabdomyoma is by far the most common primary heart tumor in children. Rhabdomyomas typically occupy the ventricular myocardium, but can also be found in the atria. Large lesions may interfere with intracardiac blood flow and in extreme cases may result in critical obstruction to the inflow or outflow tracts. The natural history of rhabdomyomas is usually spontaneous regression in early childhood, partly because of their dependence on maternal hormones. The finding of multiple rhabdomyomas essentially confirms the diagnosis of tuberous sclerosis, especially in the context of a positive family history.

Atlas of Pediatric Echocardiography. https://doi.org/10.1016/B978-0-323-75981-6.00035-2

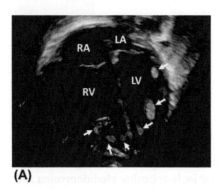 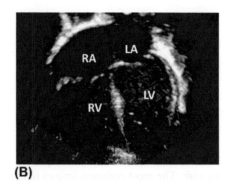

(A) **(B)**

FIGURE 1

(A) Patient with tuberous sclerosis. Apical four-chamber view showing multiple cardiac rhabdomyomas (*arrows*) involving both the right and left ventricles. The tumors vary in size. (B) Spontaneous resolution of all rhabdomyomas in the same child, which occurred several months after birth. *LA*, left atrium; *LV*, left ventricle; *RA*, right atrium; *RV*, right ventricle.

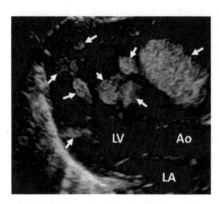

FIGURE 2

Parasternal long-axis view demonstrating a large number of rhabdomyomas (*arrows*) affecting both ventricles. Note the presence of a giant right ventricular rhabdomyoma. *Ao*, aorta; *LA*, left atrium; *LV*, left ventricle.

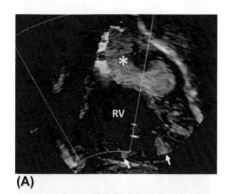

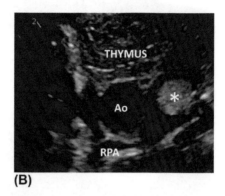

(A)

(B)

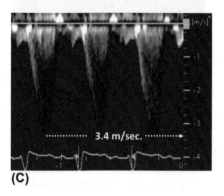

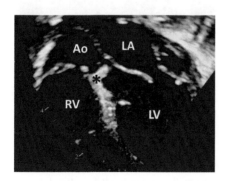

(C)

FIGURE 3

Patient with tuberous sclerosis. (A) Subcostal long-axis view illustrating a giant rhabdomyoma (*asterisk*) arising from the interventricular septum. The lesion causes significant right ventricular outflow tract (RVOT) obstruction with turbulent flow. *Arrows* indicate two smaller right ventricular rhabdomyomas. (B) Suprasternal notch view showing the proximal ascending aorta and pulmonary artery en face. In systole, the giant septal rhabdomyoma (*asterisk*) prolapses across the pulmonary valve into the pulmonary artery. (C) Continuous-wave Doppler of the RVOT from the subcostal long-axis view demonstrating turbulent flow caused by the tumor. *Ao*, aorta; *RV* right ventricle; *RPA*, right pulmonary artery.

FIGURE 4

Apical five-chamber view illustrating a relatively small rhabdomyoma (*asterisk*) arising from the outlet septum and protruding into the left ventricular outflow tract (LVOT). The tumor is more echogenic than the rest of the interventricular septum. The left ventricle is severely dilated and dysfunctional due to significant obstruction of the LVOT caused by the lesion. *Ao*, aorta; *LA*, left atrium; *LV*, left ventricle; *RV*, right ventricle.

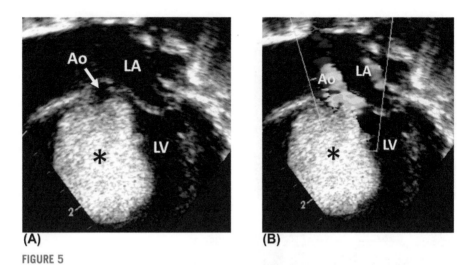

FIGURE 5

(A) Apical five-chamber view showing a giant septal rhabdomyoma (*asterisk*) causing significant left ventricular outflow tract (LVOT) obstruction. (B) Color flow Doppler demonstrating turbulent flow across the LVOT. *Ao*, aorta; *LA*, left atrium; *LV*, left ventricle.

Fibroma

Cardiac fibromas usually occur as solitary lesions in the ventricular myocardium, from which they are well delineated. Their most frequent location is the interventricular septum. Despite being benign in nature, they can grow to extreme dimensions causing obstruction to blood flow and cardiac dysfunction. Where possible, surgical debulking is performed.

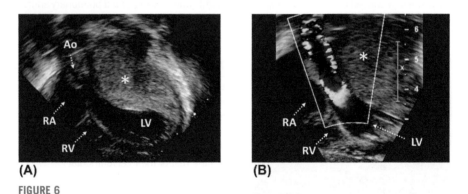

FIGURE 6

(A) Subcostal long-axis view illustrating a giant cardiac fibroma (*asterisk*) arising from the left ventricular free wall. The tumor significantly reduces the size of the left ventricular cavity. (B) Turbulent flow across the left ventricular outflow tract caused by the tumor. *LV*, left ventricle; *RA*, right atrium.

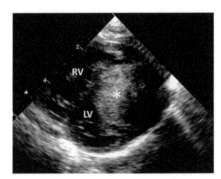

FIGURE 7

Parasternal short axis view demonstrating a large fibroma (*asterisk*) originating from the antero-septal aspect of the left ventricle. The tumor appears to be a well-defined mass in the myocardium. *LV*, left ventricle; *RV*, right ventricle.

Myxoma

Cardiac myxoma is the most common primary cardiac tumor in adults, but is relatively rare in children. It is usually found in the left atrium, attached to the interatrial septum by a short pedicle. The tumor has an irregular, lobulated, and often heterogenous appearance, and its fragments may embolize. Surgical resection is the only treatment, but if incomplete, there is a high recurrence rate.

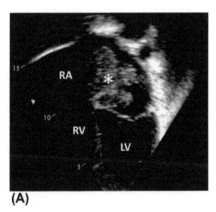
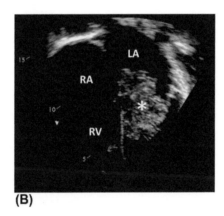

(A) **(B)**

FIGURE 8

(A) Apical four-chamber view in a child with a left atrial myxoma (*asterisk*). The tumor has an irregular and lobulated appearance with areas of hyper and hypoechogenicity creating the impression of nonhomogeneity. (B) In diastole, the tumoral mass moves across the mitral valve into the left ventricle causing severe obstruction to mitral inflow. The lesion is attached to the atrial septum by a short, broad-based pedicle. *LV*, left ventricle; *RA*, right atrium; *RV*, right ventricle.

Other tumors

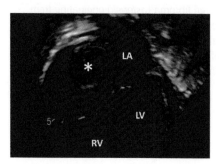

FIGURE 9

Apical four-chamber view in a patient with a primary Wilms tumor (*asterisk*). The tumor invades the inferior vena cava and right atrium. *LV*, left ventricle; *RA*, right atrium; *RV*, right ventricle.

Pulmonary hypertension

28

Pulmonary hypertension (PH) is defined by a resting mean pulmonary artery pressure ≥25 mmHg (as measured by cardiac catheterization). PH occurs in a wide range of conditions, which include idiopathic PH, PH secondary to congenital or acquired heart disease, lung disease, chronic thromboembolism, infection, and connective tissue disorders, etc.

Despite some limitations, echocardiography is a very useful tool for assessment of the pulmonary artery pressure. The systolic pulmonary artery pressure can be directly derived from the continuous wave Doppler of the tricuspid regurgitant jet by the use of the simplified Bernoulli equation. This requires measurement of the tricuspid regurgitation peak velocity along with an indirect estimation of the right atrial pressure. Similarly, the diastolic pulmonary artery pressure can be calculated using the end-diastolic pulmonary regurgitation velocity and the assumed right atrial pressure.

In the absence of tricuspid or pulmonary regurgitation, the diagnosis of PH relies on indirect echocardiographic features, which include the presence of right heart and pulmonary artery dilatation, right ventricular dysfunction and hypertrophy, flattening of the interventricular septum, or abnormal flow pattern in the pulmonary artery. However, echocardiographic screening for mild PH in asymptomatic patients remains difficult.

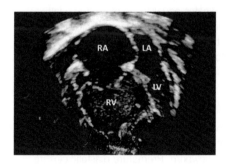

FIGURE 1

Apical four-chamber view showing severe right atrial and ventricular dilatation causing compression of the left-sided chambers. Also note the presence of significant right ventricular hypertrophy. *LA*, left atrium; *LV*, left ventricle; *RA*, right atrium; *RV*, right ventricle.

Atlas of Pediatric Echocardiography. https://doi.org/10.1016/B978-0-323-75981-6.00004-2

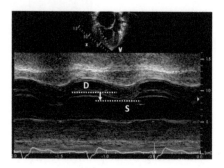

FIGURE 2

Assessment of the longitudinal right ventricular (RV) systolic function by tricuspid annular plane systolic excursion (**TAPSE**). This parameter is measured by M-mode from the apical four-chamber view. The cursor is aligned with the lateral aspect of the tricuspid annulus. TAPSE corresponds to the distance (in mm) by which the lateral tricuspid annulus moves toward the apex of the heart between end-diastole (D) and end-systole (S). The higher the value, the better the RV function. Normal reference ranges are age dependant (>7–11 mm in neonates, >15–25 mm in adults). This figure shows decreased TAPSE in a patient with severe PH and RV systolic dysfunction.

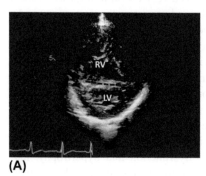

(A)

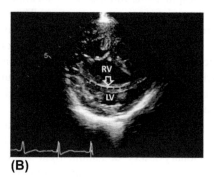

(B)

FIGURE 3

(A) Parasternal short-axis view in a child with systemic level PH. In systole, there is flattening of the interventricular septum (*black dashed line*) causing the left ventricle to become D-shaped (instead of O-shaped). This indicates equalization of right and left ventricular systolic pressures. (B) In diastole, the interventricular septum (*black dashed line*) bows into the left ventricle (*hollow arrow*) as the right ventricular diastolic pressure exceeds the left ventricular diastolic pressure. Note the right ventricular hypertrophy and dilatation. *LV*, left ventricle; *RV*, right ventricle.

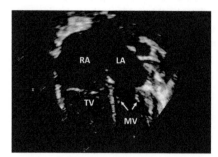

FIGURE 4

Apical four-chamber view in a neonate with persistent pulmonary hypertension of the newborn. Premature diastolic closure of the tricuspid valve occurs, while the mitral valve remains open (*arrows*). This is due to the high right ventricular diastolic pressure. *LA*, left atrium; *LV*, left ventricle; *RA*, right atrium; *RV*, right ventricle.

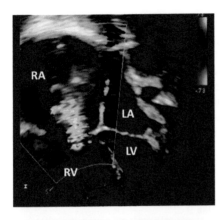

FIGURE 5

Apical four-chamber view showing severe tricuspid regurgitation in a child with end-stage PH. As a result, there is an extreme right atrial dilatation. *LA*, left atrium; *LV*, left ventricle; *RA*, right atrium; *RV*, right ventricle.

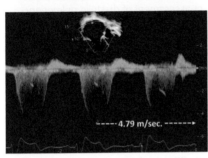

FIGURE 6

Direct assessment of systolic pulmonary artery pressure from continuous-wave Doppler of the tricuspid regurgitation (TR). The systolic pressure gradient between the right ventricle (RV) and the right atrium (RA) is proportional to the TR peak velocity. Using the simplified Bernoulli equation (see below), the systolic pulmonary artery pressure is obtained by adding the value of the assumed RA pressure to the value of the measured RV-RA systolic gradient. This figure shows significantly elevated TR peak velocity in a patient with severe PH.

Systolic RV pressure − RA pressure $= 4 \times$ (TR peak velocity in m/s)^2

Systolic PA pressure = systolic RV pressure $= 4 \times$ (TR peak velocity)$^2 +$ RA pressure

Systolic PA pressure $= 4 \times (4.79 \text{ m/s})^2 + 15 \text{ mmHg} = \underline{106.7 \text{ mmHg}}$

[assumed RA pressure $= 15$ mmHg]

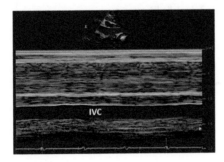

FIGURE 7

Semiquantitative assessment of the right atrial pressure based on the evaluation of the diameter and the inspiratory collapsibility of the inferior vena cava (IVC) on subcostal M-mode. Unlike in adults, age-matched IVC dimensions have not been well defined in children. More than 50% inspiratory collapse of the IVC suggests a right atrial pressure that is <10 mmHg. This figure shows a severely dilated IVC with no respiratory variation in IVC diameter indicating an RA pressure >10–15 mmHg.

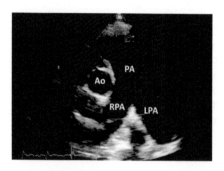

FIGURE 8

Parasternal short-axis view demonstrating a dilated pulmonary artery in a patient with severe PH. Note the difference between the size of the aorta and the pulmonary artery. *Ao*, aorta; *LPA*, left pulmonary artery; *PA*, pulmonary artery; *RPA*, right pulmonary artery.

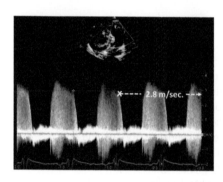

FIGURE 9

Direct assessment of diastolic pulmonary artery (PA) pressure from continuous wave Doppler of pulmonary regurgitation (PR). The diastolic PA pressure is calculated analogously to the systolic PA pressure (see Figure 6 for explanation). For the purposes of the calculation, the right ventricular end-diastolic pressure (RV) is considered to be equal to the right atrial pressure (RA). This figure shows an example of a significant elevation of the end-diastolic PR velocity in a child with severe PH.

$$\text{Diastolic PA pressure} = 4 \times (\text{end-diastolic PR velocity})^2 + \text{RV diastolic pressure}$$
$$= 4 \times (\text{end-diastolic PR velocity})^2 + \text{RA pressure}$$
$$= 4 \times \left(2.8 \text{ m/s}\right)^2 + 10 \text{ mmHg} = 31.3 + 10 = \underline{41.3 \text{ mmHg}}$$

[PR velocity 2.8 m/s (*white arrow*), assumed RA pressure 10 mmHg]

Systolic PA pressure $= 4 \times (\text{peak TR velocity in m/s})^2 +$ assumed RA pressure

Diastolic PA pressure $= 4 \times (\text{end-diastolic PR velocity in m/s})^2 +$ assumed RA pressure

Mean PA pressure $= 1/3$ systolic PA pressure $+ 2/3$ diastolic PA pressure

PA, pulmonary artery; *PR*, pulmonary regurgitation; *RA*, right atrium; *TR*, tricuspid regurgitation

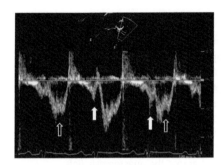

FIGURE 10

Continuous-wave Doppler of the right ventricular outflow tract (RVOT) demonstrating mid-systolic notching (*hollow arrows*) in the RVOT envelope. This flow pattern is typically seen in patients with severely elevated pulmonary vascular resistance. Plain arrows indicate antegrade end-diastolic flow in the pulmonary artery caused by right atrial contraction, a feature that is consistent with diastolic dysfunction of the right ventricle.

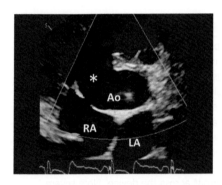

FIGURE 11

The presence of a ventricular septal defect (VSD) makes it possible to evaluate the systolic pressure gradient between the aorta and the pulmonary artery. This figure shows the parasternal short-axis view of a large perimembranous VSD (*asterisk*) in a child with Eisenmenger syndrome. There is a systolic right-to-left shunt across the defect consistent with suprasystemic pulmonary artery pressure. *Ao*, aorta; *LA*, left atrium; *RA*, right atrium.

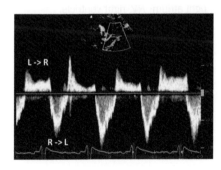

FIGURE 12

Continuous-wave Doppler of ductal flow from the parasternal short-axis view in a neonate with persistent pulmonary hypertension of the newborn (PPHN). The systolic and diastolic aortic to pulmonary arterial pressure gradients can be assessed from the Doppler waveform, which in this example shows a low-velocity bidirectional shunt. In systole, the pulmonary artery pressure becomes suprasystemic (right-to-left systolic shunt, R→L), while in diastole the shunt reverses (left-to-right diastolic shunt, L→R).

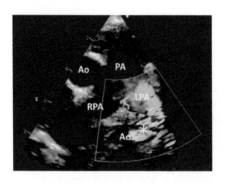

FIGURE 13

The treatment of some patients with suprasystemic PH consists of creating a Potts shunt, a side-to-side anastomosis between the left pulmonary artery and the descending aorta (*asterisk*). This procedure preserves the right ventricular (RV) function by relieving the increased RV afterload. Note the systolic right-to-left shunt across the anastomosis (left pulmonary artery→aorta). *Ao,* aorta; *LPA,* left pulmonary artery; *PA,* pulmonary artery; *RPA,* right pulmonary artery.

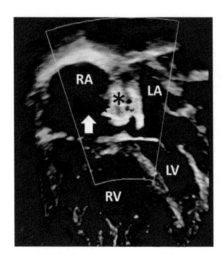

FIGURE 14

Apical four-chamber view demonstrating an implantable atrial flow regulator (*asterisk*). This device is implanted in selected patients with severe PH, whom it creates a small interatrial communication. It allows bidirectional shunting at atrial level and improves clinical symptoms by decompressing the right atrium. In this example, there is a left-to-right shunt (*arrow*) across the device. Note severe right ventricular hypertrophy and dilatation. *LA,* left atrium; *LV,* left ventricle; *RA,* right atrium; *RV,* right ventricle.

Common genetic disorders associated with heart disease

29

Echocardiographic screening in patients with genetic disease plays an important role in daily practice. Early detection of possible cardiac complications is essential and enables prompt treatment. Some disorders have very typical echocardiographic features. This chapter describes some of the most common genetic disorders associated with heart disease.

Williams syndrome

Williams syndrome is caused by a heterozygous deletion of a specific region of chromosome seven that contains, among others, the elastin gene. Affected patients have distinctive facial features, learning difficulties, and loose skin due to the reduced deposition of elastin. Cardiac abnormalities are present in the vast majority of cases and typically include supravalvar aortic stenosis, diffuse aortic hypoplasia, and stenotic lesions affecting the proximal and distal pulmonary arterial tree. Some patients also experience coronary artery involvement.

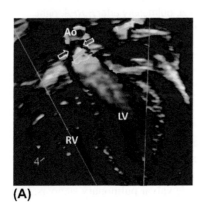
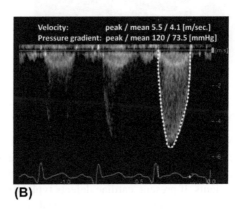

(A)   **(B)**

FIGURE 1

(A) Zoomed apical five-chamber view in a child with Williams syndrome and supravalvar aortic stenosis (*white arrows*). Note the flow turbulence starting at the level of the narrowed sinotubular junction. (B) Same patient. Continuous-wave Doppler of the left ventricular outflow tract showing a significantly increased blood flow velocity of 5.5 m/s, consistent with a severe degree of stenosis. *Ao*, aorta; *RV*, right ventricle; *LV*, left ventricle.

Atlas of Pediatric Echocardiography. https://doi.org/10.1016/B978-0-323-75981-6.00023-6

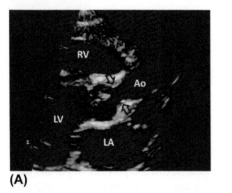
(A)

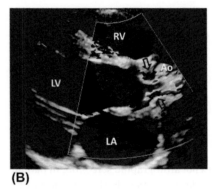
(B)

FIGURE 2

(A) Zoomed parasternal long-axis view in a patient with Williams syndrome. There is a discrete supravalvar aortic stenosis (*black arrows*) with normal caliber ascending aorta. This creates an "hourglass" appearance. (B) Corresponding color flow mapping demonstrating turbulent flow across the sinotubular junction. *Ao*, aorta; *LA*, left atrium; *LV*, left ventricle; *RV*, right ventricle.

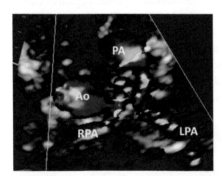

FIGURE 3

Zoomed left subclavicular view in a patient with Williams syndrome illustrating severely hypoplastic branch pulmonary arteries with turbulent flow on color flow mapping. *Ao*, aorta; *LPA*, left pulmonary artery; *PA*, pulmonary artery; *RPA*, right pulmonary artery.

Noonan syndrome

Noonan syndrome has been associated with mutations in a number of genes. From a clinical point of view, the syndrome is characterized by facial dysmorphism, short stature, and chest deformities, but the phenotypic expression varies widely among patients. If present, cardiac defects typically include valvar pulmonary stenosis, hypertrophic cardiomyopathy, and atrial septal defects.

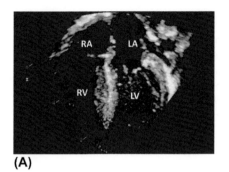
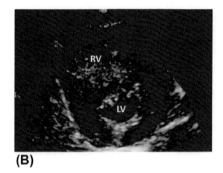

(A) **(B)**

FIGURE 4

(A) Hypertrophic cardiomyopathy in a child with Noonan syndrome seen from the apical four-chamber view. (B) Same heart shown from the parasternal short-axis view. *LA*, left atrium; *LV*, left ventricle; *RA*, right atrium; *RV*, right ventricle.

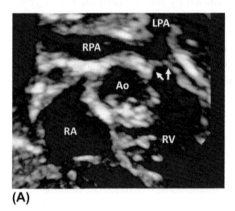
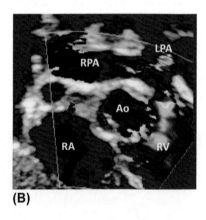

(A) **(B)**

FIGURE 5

(A) Subcostal short-axis view in a patient with Noonan syndrome and valvar pulmonary stenosis. There are thickening and doming (*white arrows*) of the leaflets. (B) Color flow mapping demonstrating turbulent flow across the valve. *Ao*, aorta; *LPA*, left pulmonary artery; *RA*, right atrium; *RPA*, right pulmonary artery; *RV*, right ventricle.

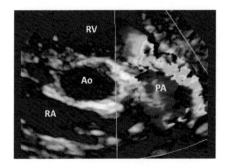

FIGURE 6

Zoomed parasternal short axis view with color flow mapping of the right ventricular outflow tract illustrating valvar pulmonary stenosis. There is turbulent flow across the valve and poststenotic dilatation of the pulmonary artery with swirling blood flow. *Ao*, aorta; *PA*, pulmonary artery; *RA*, right atrium; *RV*, right ventricle.

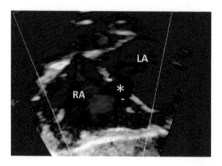

FIGURE 7

Child with Noonan syndrome. Ostium secundum atrial septal defect (*asterisk*) seen from the subcostal short-axis view. There is a left-to-right shunt across the defect on color flow mapping. *LA*, left atrium; *RA*, right atrium.

Marfan syndrome

Marfan syndrome is a multisystemic connective tissue disorder affecting the heart, blood vessels, eyes, spine, and chest. It is caused by mutations in the FBN1 gene, coding for the fibrillin-1 protein. From a cardiac point of view, the hallmark of the disease is aortic root dilatation, which may be complicated by aortic dissection. Pulmonary artery dilatation is rare as the pressure is much lower in the pulmonary artery compared to the aorta. Mitral valve prolapse represents another common feature associated with the syndrome. Tricuspid valve involvement may also occur in severe neonatal forms of the disease.

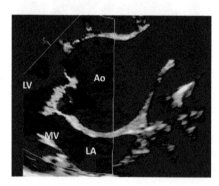

FIGURE 8

Zoomed parasternal long-axis view in a patient with Marfan syndrome and extreme aortic root dilatation. Note the presence of moderate aortic regurgitation due to the dilatation of the aortic annulus. *Ao*, aorta; *LA*, left atrium; *LV*, left ventricle; *MV*, mitral valve.

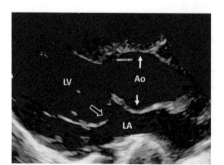

FIGURE 9

Neonatal form of Marfan syndrome with aortic root dilatation (*white arrows*) and mitral valve prolapse (*hollow arrow*), demonstrated from the parasternal long-axis view. *Ao*, aorta; *LA*, left atrium; *LV*, left ventricle.

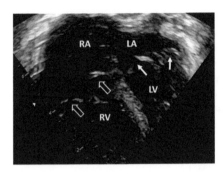

FIGURE 10

Apical four-chamber view illustrating significant prolapse of the mitral (*white arrows*) and tricuspid valves (*hollow arrows*) in an infant with severe Marfan syndrome. *LA*, left atrium; *LV*, left ventricle; *RA*, right atrium; *RV*, right ventricle.

Turner syndrome

Turner syndrome is caused by a partial or complete loss of one of the two X chromosomes and therefore only affects women. From a clinical point of view, the syndrome is characterized by a broad chest, wide neck, low-set ears, low hairline, edema in hands and feet (particularly in neonates), and slow growth. Approximately one-third of the patients with Turner syndrome have a bicommissural (bicuspid) aortic valve or develop coarctation of the aorta.

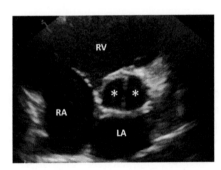

FIGURE 11

Zoomed parasternal short-axis view in a patient with Turner syndrome and bicommissural ("purely" bicuspid) aortic valve. Each cusp is marked with an *asterisk*. *LA*, left atrium; *RA*, right atrium; *RV*, right ventricle.

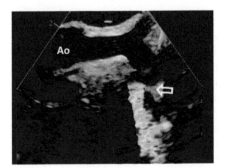

FIGURE 12

Suprasternal notch view demonstrating coarctation of the aorta (Ao) in a neonate with Turner syndrome. The *hollow arrow* indicates the coarctation shelf.

Down syndrome

Congenital heart defects occur in approximately half of the children with trisomy 21 and are a major cause of early-life mortality and morbidity. Defects of the atrioventricular septum, encountered in approximately one-third of the patients, represent by far the most common cardiac diagnosis. Atrial or ventricular septal defects, patent ductus arteriosus, and tetralogy of Fallot account for the majority of the remaining defects.

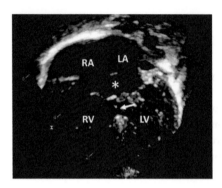

FIGURE 13

Apical four-chamber view in a child with trisomy 21 and complete atrio-ventricular septal defect. *Asterisk* indicates the ostium primum atrial septal defect, *white arrow* the inlet ventricular septal defect. Note the presence of a common atrio-ventricular valve. *LA*, left atrium; *LV*, left ventricle; *RA*, right atrium; *RV*, right ventricle.

DiGeorge syndrome

DiGeorge syndrome, also known as 22q11 deletion syndrome, is characterized by distinctive facial features and thymic and parathyroid hypoplasia, resulting in immunodeficiency and hypocalcemia. Cardiac defects are not uncommon and typically affect the ventricular outflow tracts. The most common cardiac diagnoses include interrupted aortic arch and truncus arteriosus. Tetralogy of Fallot, double-outlet right ventricle, or large ventricular septal defects may also occur.

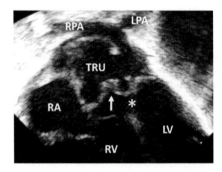

FIGURE 14

Zoomed apical five-chamber view in a patient with DiGeorge syndrome and type 1 persistent truncus arteriosus. The truncal valve (*arrow*) is dysplastic, has thickened leaflets and overrides the ventricular septal defect (*asterisk*). Note the origin of the pulmonary artery from the truncus. *LPA*, left pulmonary artery; *LV*, left ventricle; *RA*, right atrium; *RPA*, right pulmonary artery; *RV*, right ventricle; *TRU*, truncus.

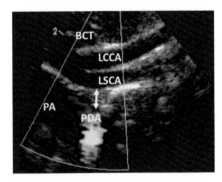

FIGURE 15

Suprasternal notch view showing aortic arch interruption distal to the left subclavian artery (type A). The *double arrow* marks the interrupted segment. Color flow mapping demonstrating diastolic flow reversal in the duct. *BCT*, brachiocephalic trunk; *LCCA*, left common carotid artery; *LSCA*, left subclavian artery; *PA*, pulmonary artery; *PDA*, patent ductus arteriosus.

Glycogen storage diseases

Glycogen storage diseases are metabolic disorders characterized by abnormal glycogen synthesis or breakdown. This results in an accumulation of glycogen in the skeletal muscles, causing generalized hypotonia. Myocardial involvement may also occur, leading to the development of cardiomyopathy. Enzyme replacement therapy is the only treatment available in some cases.

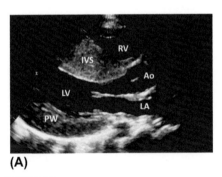
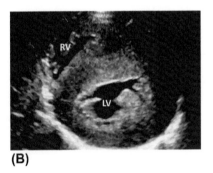

(A)   **(B)**

FIGURE 16

(A) Parasternal long-axis view in a toddler with Pompe disease and hypertrophic cardiomyopathy. There is severe hypertrophy of the interventricular septum and the left ventricular posterior wall. (B) Same heart seen from the parasternal short-axis view. *Ao*, aorta; *IVS*, interventricular septum; *LA*, left atrium; *LV*, left ventricle; *PW*, posterior wall; *RV*, right ventricle.

Mechanical circulatory support and heart transplantation

30

Mechanical circulatory support

Despite recent progress in medical therapy, children with end-stage heart failure have limited treatment options. **Mechanical circulatory support** is used as a bridge to heart transplantation or recovery, in those patients who are refractory to maximal medical therapy. **ECMO** (Extra Corporeal Membrane Oxygenation) is the most common type of support in the pediatric population, allowing immediate biventricular and respiratory assistance. Use is typically limited to less than 2–3 weeks.

Lack of organ donors and the long waiting times have stimulated the development of long-term ventricular assist devices, such as Berlin Heart™ or Heart Ware™. Their use can exceed 1 year. Berlin Heart™ is an air-driven pulsatile flow device with an external pump. It can either support solely the left ventricle or provide biventricular support. Heart Ware™ is an internal pump located in the pericardial space. Unlike Berlin Heart™, it is a continuous-flow device.

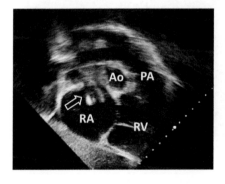

FIGURE 1

Subcostal short-axis view in a patient with veno-arterial (VA) ECMO. Deoxygenated blood is sucked into the ECMO circuit from a venous cannula, the tip of which is typically located in the right atrium. After oxygenation, blood is returned to the body via an arterial cannula (not shown), usually inserted into the right common carotid artery. *Ao*, aorta; *PA*, pulmonary artery; *RA*, right atrium; *RV*, right ventricle.

Atlas of Pediatric Echocardiography. https://doi.org/10.1016/B978-0-323-75981-6.00032-7

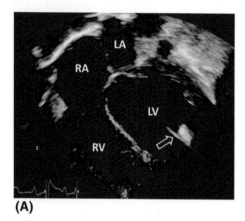
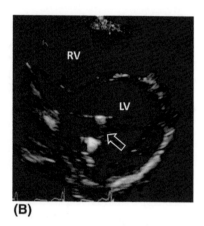

(A) **(B)**

FIGURE 2

(A) Patient with dilated cardiomyopathy. Apical four-chamber view demonstrating a Heart Ware™ device inflow cannula (*hollow arrow*) inserted into the apex of the left ventricle. The cannula is connected to a pump, which then returns the blood back to the aorta via an outflow cannula (not shown). (B) Heart Ware™ device inflow cannula (*hollow arrow*) seen from the parasternal short-axis view. *LA*, left atrium; *LV*, left ventricle; *RA*, right atrium; *RV*, right ventricle.

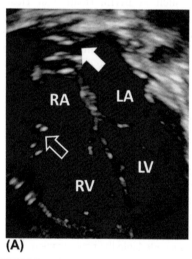
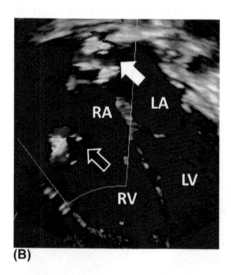

(A) **(B)**

FIGURE 3

In children with restrictive cardiomyopathy, the ventricles are usually too small to accommodate a large cannula. However, severe atrial dilatation, typically present in this condition, provides enough space for atrial cannulation. (A) Patient with restrictive cardiomyopathy and biventricular support by two Berlin Heart™ pumps. Apical four-chamber view illustrating left atrial (*white arrow*) and right atrial (*hollow arrow*) inflow cannulae. (B) Color flow mapping demonstrating flow across the cannulae. *LA*, left atrium; *LV*, left ventricle; *RA*, right atrium; *RV*, right ventricle.

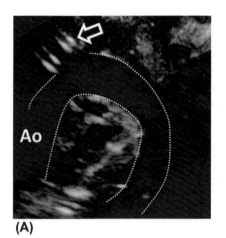
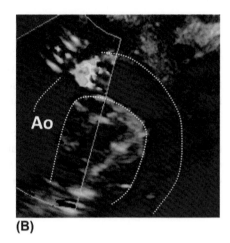

(A)   **(B)**

FIGURE 4

Suprasternal notch view in a child with a Berlin Heart™. (A) The *dotted lines* indicate the outline of the aortic arch. Note the presence of an aortic outflow cannula (*hollow arrow*). (B) Color flow mapping showing blood flow through the cannula to the aorta (Ao).

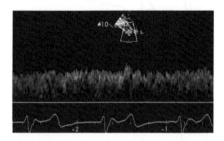

FIGURE 5

Continuous-wave Doppler interrogation of the descending aorta from the subcostal approach demonstrating a continuous flow pattern. Patients supported by a continuous-flow device (such as ECMO or Heart Ware™) and no spontaneous left ventricular ejection, will have continuous flow in the aorta.

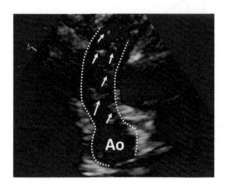

FIGURE 6

Suprasternal notch view showing a detail of the ascending aorta (Ao). There is thrombus formation in the Heart Ware™ device pump (not shown) due to an infection. Note the spontaneous echo contrast (*arrows*) in the aorta, generated by the increased friction inside the pump.

Heart transplantation

Heart transplantation has become an accepted therapy for end-stage heart failure with approximately 500 heart transplants performed each year in children around the world. The survival rate has increased considerably with advances in surgical technique, postoperative care, and immunosuppression. In most cases, it can reach 15–20 years.

The overall prognosis in transplant recipients is largely determined by complications including primary graft failure, acute rejection, and coronary allograft vasculopathy. Apart from changes in cardiac function, echocardiographic recognition is often difficult and relies solely on the presence of nonspecific features.

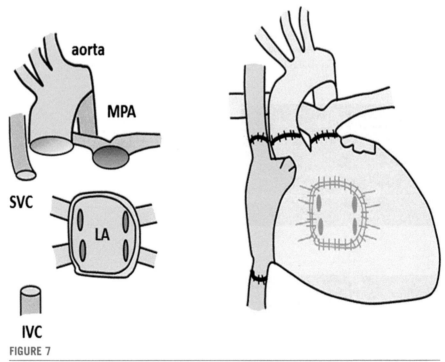

FIGURE 7

Orthotopic heart transplantation is most commonly performed using the bicaval technique. The heart of the recipient is removed, leaving only a left atrial cuff with the pulmonary vein orifices. Donor heart is then implanted and the left atrial, IVC, SVC, aortic, and pulmonary anastomoses are carried out. *IVC*, inferior vena cava; *LA*, left atrium; *PA*, pulmonary artery; *SVC*, superior vena cava.

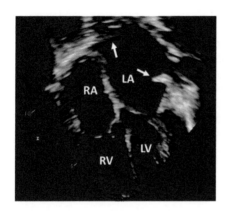

FIGURE 8

Apical four-chamber view in a heart transplant recipient. The *arrows* indicate the anastomosis between the left atrial cuff of the recipient and the donor heart. *LA*, left atrium; *LV*, left ventricle; *RA*, right atrium; *RV*, right ventricle.

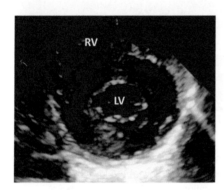

FIGURE 9

Parasternal short-axis view demonstrating left ventricular pseudohypertrophy. Pediatric heart transplant recipients typically receive organs from older donors to ensure adequate long-term cardiac output. This results in the appearance of ventricular pseudohypertrophy. *LV*, left ventricle; *RV*, right ventricle.

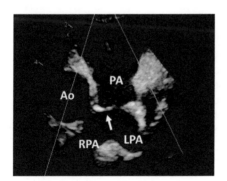

FIGURE 10

Zoomed parasternal short-axis view. Pulmonary anastomosis (*arrow*) between the donor heart and the native pulmonary artery. *Ao*, aorta; *LPA*, left pulmonary artery; *PA*, pulmonary artery; *RPA*, right pulmonary artery.

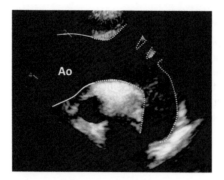

FIGURE 11

Aortic anastomosis visualized from the suprasternal notch view. Note the significant difference between the size of the aorta in the donor heart (*solid line*) (Ao) and the native aorta of the recipient (*dotted line*). This is due to the size mismatch between the two organs.

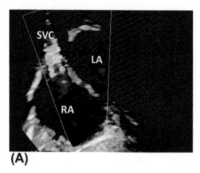

(A)

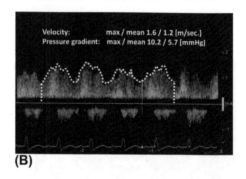

(B)

FIGURE 12

(A) Stenotic superior vena cava (SVC) anastomosis visualized from a zoomed subcostal short-axis view. Color flow mapping demonstrating turbulent flow at the level of the anastomosis. (B) Continuous-wave Doppler interrogation of the SVC demonstrates a mean gradient across the anastomosis of 5.7 mmHg with flow not returning to baseline. *LA*, left atrium; *RA*, right atrium.

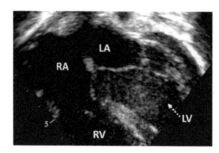

FIGURE 13

Heart transplant recipient on ECMO support due to severe primary graft failure. The left ventricle is dilated, dysfunctional, and filled with spontaneous echo contrast. Note the hyperechogenicity of the left ventricular myocardium. *LA*, left atrium; *LV*, left ventricle; *RA*, right atrium; *RV*, right ventricle.

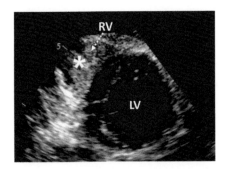

FIGURE 14

Primary graft failure in an ECMO assisted heart transplant recipient. Note the extensive right ventricular thrombus (*asterisk*), which occurred in the context of severe biventricular dysfunction. The patient required a subsequent urgent heart retransplantation. *LV*, left ventricle; *RV*, right ventricle.

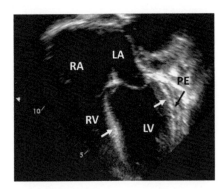

FIGURE 15

Apical four-chamber view in a child with severely impaired left ventricular function due to acute allograft rejection. The left ventricular myocardium is diffusely swollen and hyperechogenic (*white arrows*). There is a small pericardial effusion, which is often present in these cases (*black arrow*). *LA*, left atrium; *LV*, left ventricle; *PE*, pericardial effusion; *RA*, right atrium; *RV*, right ventricle.

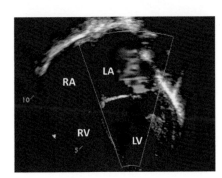

FIGURE 16

Cardiac allograft vasculopathy is the leading long-term cause of graft failure. It is characterized by the progressive development of diffuse intimal hyperplasia of the coronary artery tree. This patient developed left ventricular dysfunction with severe mitral regurgitation due to significant left coronary artery involvement. *LA*, left atrium; *LV*, left ventricle; *RA*, right atrium; *RV*, right ventricle.

Index

'*Note*: Page numbers followed by "f" indicate figures and "t" indicate tables.'

A

Aberrant left subclavian artery, 150f, 191, 192f, 196f
Aberrant right subclavian artery, 152f–153f, 191, 197f
Absent pulmonary valve syndrome, 109f, 121, 130, 130f–131f
Acute allograft rejection, 286, 289f
Acute coronary artery thrombosis, 237, 239f
Acute pericarditis, 253, 254f–255f
Acute rheumatic carditis, 241, 241f
ALCAPA. *See* Anomalous Left Coronary Artery from the Pulmonary Artery (ALCAPA)
Anomalous Left Coronary Artery from the Pulmonary Artery (ALCAPA), 211, 211f–213f
Anomalous origin of the left main coronary artery from the right coronary cusp, 214f
Anomalous origin of the right coronary artery from the left coronary cusp, 215f
Aortic annulus, 20f
Aortic arch hypoplasia, 157f, 184f, 188
Aortic atresia, 155, 157f
Aortic overriding, 102f, 121, 124f–125f
Aortic regurgitation, 92, 97f–98f, 241, 244f
Aortic root, 20f, 278, 278f
Aortic stenosis
    subvalvar, 89, 90f–91f, 188, 189f
    supravalvar, 99, 99f–100f, 275f–276f
    valvar, 92, 92f–97f
Aortic valve
    bicommissural, 92, 95f, 181, 279, 279f
    prolapse, 57f, 60f, 97f
    tricommissural, 92f, 95f
    unicommissural, 94f, 96f
Aorto-pulmonary window, 179, 179f–180f
Apical views 9, 9f–12f
Arterial switch operation, 117, 133, 139f
Ascending aorta (dilatation), 96f, 278f
ASD. *See* Atrial septal defect (ASD)
Atrial morphology, 29–31, 30f–32f
Atrial septal defect (ASD), 45, 46f–52f
    coronary sinus defect, 45, 46f, 52f
    ostium primum, 45, 46f, 50f, 63, 67f–68f, 70f, 161f,
    ostium secundum, 45, 46f–49f, 50f, 278f
    patch closure, 52f, 70f, 247f
    sinus venosus, 45, 46f, 51f
Atrial situs, 29–31, 30f–32f
    inversus, 29, 30f–32f
    solitus, 29, 30f–32f
Atrio-ventricular connection
    biventricular, 33, 33f–34f, 36
    mode of, 36, 36f–37f
    univentricular, 34, 35f, 36, 155
Atrio-ventricular discordance, 37f, 141, 141f
Atrio-ventricular septal defect, 63, 64f–70f
    complete, 37f, 63, 64f–66f, 69f–70f
    partial, 63, 64f, 67f–68f, 70f
    transitional, 63, 64f, 66f–67f
    unbalanced, 65f, 66f, 155, 161, 161f
Atrio-ventricular valve offset, 32, 34f, 144f
AVSD, Atrio-ventricular septal defect (AVSD)

B

Balloon atrial septostomy, 133, 138f, 169f
BCPA. *See* Bidirectional cavo-pulmonary anastomosis (BCPA)
Berlin Heart, 283, 284f–285f
Bicommissural (bicuspid) aortic valve, 92, 95f, 181, 279, 279f
Bicuspid (bicommissural) aortic valve, 92, 95f, 181, 279, 279f
Bidirectional cavo-pulmonary anastomosis (BCPA), 169, 171f
Biplane (Simpson's) method, 21f
Branch pulmonary arteries, 16f, 20f, 147, 150f
    hypoplasia, 128f, 276f

C

Cardiac allograft vasculopathy, 289f
Cardiac position, 28, 28f–29f
Cardiac tumors 263–268
    fibroma, 266, 266f–267f
    myxoma, 75f, 267, 267f
    rhabdomyoma, 263, 264f–266f
    Wilms tumor, 268f
Cardiomyopathy
    dilated (DCM), 79f, 221, 225, 226f–227f, 284f
    hypertrophic, 89, 91f, 225, 228f–231f, 281f
    noncompaction, 225, 236, 236f
    restrictive, 225, 232f–236f, 256, 259, 260f, 262t

CCTGA. *See* Congenitally Corrected Transposition of the Great Arteries (CCTGA)
Coarctation of the aorta, 181, 182f–187f, 279, 279f
Color flow mapping (CFM), 3
Common atrio-ventricular (AV) valve, 63, 64f–70f, 168f, 280f
Common collector vein, 200f–202f
Complete AVSD, 37f, 63, 64f–66f, 69f–70f
Cone procedure, 88f
Confluens of pulmonary veins, 200f–201f, 203f
Congenitally corrected transposition of the great arteries (CCTGA), 34f, 141, 141f–146f
Constrictive pericarditis, 253, 259f–261f, 262t
Continuous-wave Doppler, 23
Conus
    subaortic, 111, 113f–114f, 116f
    subpulmonary, 111, 114f, 116f
Coronary aneurysm, 237, 237f–238f
Coronary artery fistula, 211, 213f, 214f
Coronary artery thrombosis, 237, 239f
Coronary sinus defect, 45, 46f, 52f
Coronary sinusoids, 159, 159f–160f
Cor triatriatum sinister, 199, 205f–206f
Criss-cross heart, 118f

D

Damus-Kaye-Stansel procedure, 169, 170f
DCM. *See* Dilated cardiomyopathy (DCM)
Deceleration time, 24f, 234f, 262t
Dextrocardia, 28, 28f–29f, 141
Diastolic flow reversal in abdominal aorta, 152f, 177f
DiGeorge syndrome, 188, 280
Dilated cardiomyopathy (DCM), 79f, 221, 225, 226f–227f, 284f
Discordance atrio-ventricular, 37f, 141, 141f
Discordance ventriculo-arterial, 41f, 133, 133f–139f, 141, 142f–143f, 162, 165f, 168f–169f
Dog leg sign, 243f
DORV. *See* Double Outlet Right Ventricle (DORV)
Double aortic arch, 191, 192f–195f
    with distal left arch atresia, 194f–195f
Double-chambered right ventricle, 101, 103f
Double inlet ventricle, 34, 155, 165, 166f–169f
    with common atrio-ventricular valve, 167f–168f
Double orifice mitral valve, 71, 72f
Double outlet right ventricle (DORV), 111, 112f–119f
    tetralogy of Fallot type, 115f, 119f

transposition type, 115f–117f
Double switch operation, 141, 146f
Down syndrome, 63, 280
dP/dt, 227f
Ductal stenting, 178f

E

Ebstein's anomaly, 81, 84f–88f
ECMO, Extra Corporeal Membrane Oxygenation (ECMO)
Endocardial fibroelastosis, 155, 156f–157f
Extra Corporeal Membrane Oxygenation, 283, 283f
Extracorporeal membrane oxygenation (ECMO), 283, 283f

F

Fenestrated fossa ovalis, 48f
Fibroma, 266, 266f–267f
Fibromuscular shelf, 89, 90f
Floating heart, 254f, 257f
Functionally single ventricle, 155–172
    double inlet ventricle, 34, 155, 165, 166f–169f
    Glenn shunt, 169, 171f
    hypoplastic left heart syndrome, 155, 156f–158f, 170f–171f, 181
    pulmonary atresia, 158, 159f–160f
    total cavo-pulmonary connection (TCPC), 169, 171f–172f
    tricuspid atresia, 35f, 81, 155, 162, 162f–165f
    unbalanced atrio-ventricular septal defect, 161, 161f
Fused commissures, 92f, 96f

G

Genetic disorders
    DiGeorge syndrome, 188, 280
    Down syndrome, 63, 280
    Glycogen storage diseases, 281, 281f
    Marfan syndrome, 278, 278f–279f
    Noonan syndrome, 276, 277f–278f
    Turner syndrome, 279, 279f
    Williams syndrome, 99f, 100f, 275, 275f–276f
Glenn shunt, 169, 171f
Glycogen storage diseases, 281, 281f

H

HCM. *See* Hypertrophic cardiomyopathy (HCM)
Heart transplantation, 283, 286f–289f
Heart Ware device, 283, 284f–285f
Hemitruncus, 153f
Hemopericardium, 258f

Hepatic veins, systolic flow reversal, 23f, 84f, 260f, 262t
Homograft, 154f
Hypertrophic cardiomyopathy (HCM), 89, 91f, 225, 228f–231f, 281f
  systolic anterior motion (SAM), 89, 91f, 228, 230f–231f
Hypoplastic left heart syndrome, 155, 156f–158f, 170f–171f, 181

I

Infective endocarditis (IE), 247–251
  aortic valve, 250f
  mitral valve, 247f–248f
  pulmonary valve, 251f
  tricuspid valve, 249f
Inferior vena cava (IVC), 5f, 7f, 31, 207f, 209f, 271f
Infundibular septum, 53, 54f, 55f, 59f–60f, 89, 111, 112f
  anterior deviation, 58f, 101, 102f, 115f, 121, 122f
  posterior deviation, 58f, 89, 91f, 115f, 135f–136f, 188, 189f
Inlet VSD, 53, 63, 64f–65f, 82f, 118f, 144f, 161f
Interrupted aortic arch, 91f, 152f–153f, 188, 188f–189f, 281f
Isolated cleft of the anterior mitral valve leaflet, 71, 73f
Isomerism
  left atrial, 27, 29, 30f, 32f, 65f, 207, 209f
  right atrial, 29, 30f, 32f, 66f, 161f

K

Kawasaki disease, 237, 237f–240f
Kommerell diverticulum, 192f, 196f

L

Left anterior descending coronary artery (LAD), 16f, 20f, 212f, 215f–216f, 238f–239f
Left aortic arch with aberrant right subclavian artery, 191, 197f
Left atrial appendage, 30f
Left coronary artery, 16f, 20f, 211, 211f–217f
Left circumflex coronary artery (LCx), 20f, 212f, 216f, 238f–239f
Left main coronary artery (LMCA), 16f, 20f, 212f, 237f, 239f
Left pulmonary artery, 16f, 19f–20f
  sling, 191, 192f, 198f
Left subclavian artery, 17f, 197f
Left superior vena cava (LSVC), 207, 207f–208f
Left ventricular hypertrophy, 89, 93f–94f, 185f, 228, 228f–229f, 281f, 287f

Left ventricular outflow tract (LVOT), 89
  aortic valve disease, 92, 92f–98f
  subvalvar aortic stenosis, 89, 90f–91f, 188, 189f
  supravalvar aortic stenosis 99, 99f–100f, 275f–276f
Levoatrial cardinal vein, 207, 207f–208f
Levocardia, 28, 28f–29f

M

Major aorto-pulmonary collaterals (MAPCAs), 127, 128f–129f
Malalignment VSD, 53, 58f, 91f, 121, 188
MAPCA. *See* Major aorto-pulmonary collaterals (MAPCA)
Marfan syndrome 278, 278f–279f
Mechanical circulatory support
  Berlin Heart, 283, 284f–285f
  Extracorporeal Membrane Oxygenation (ECMO), 283, 283f
  Heart Ware device, 283, 284f–285f
Mesocardia, 28, 28f–29f
Mitral annulus, 19f
Mitral atresia, 76f, 155, 157f,
Mitral regurgitation, 71, 73f, 78f–79f, 211f, 223f, 230f, 243f–244f, 248f, 289f
Mitral stenosis, 71, 74f–78f, 241, 242f–245f
Mitral valve
  prolapse, 71, 71f–72f, 278, 278f–279f
  prosthetic, 79f
  straddling, 36, 37f, 71, 75f
M-mode echocardiography, 22, 22f–23f
Modified Blalock-Taussig shunt, 129f, 169
Morphological right ventricle, 27, 32–33, 34f, 38, 141, 141f–146f
Motion mode (M-mode), 22, 22f–23f
Mural thrombus, 227f
Muscular VSD, 53, 54f, 57f, 60f–61f
Myocarditis, 221, 221f–223f
Myxoma, 75f, 267, 267f

N

Noncompaction cardiomyopathy, 236, 236f
Noonan syndrome, 276, 277f–278f
Normal echocardiogram, 3–26

O

Ostium primum atrial septal defect, 45, 46f, 50f, 63, 67f–68f, 70f, 161f
Ostium secundum atrial septal defect, 45, 46f–49f, 50f, 278f
Overriding aorta, 102f, 121, 124f–125f

P

Parachute mitral valve, 71, 76f–77f
Parasternal views 12, 13f–17f
Parasternal long-axis view, 13f
Parasternal short-axis view, 15f
Partial anomalous pulmonary venous connection
  (PAPVC), 199, 204f–205f
Partial AVSD, 63, 64f, 67f–68f, 70f
Patent ductus arteriosus (PDA), 129f, 153f, 158f,
  173, 174f–180f, 188f–189f, 197f,
  stenting, 178f
  reverse orientation, 129f, 174f
Patent foramen ovale, 45, 46f–47f
Pericardial disease 253, 254f–262f
  acute pericarditis, 253, 254f–255f
  cardiac tamponade, 253, 256, 257f–258f, 262t
  constrictive pericarditis, 253, 259f–261f, 262t
  postoperative hemopericardium, 258f
Pericardial effusion, 253, 254f–255f
Perimembranous VSD, 53, 54f–57f, 97f, 102f, 273f
Persistent pulmonary hypertension of the newborn
  (PPHN), 176f–177f, 273f
Persistent truncus arteriosus (PTA) 38, 40f, 147,
  148f–154f
  type I 148f, 149f
  type II 150f
  type III 150f
Perivascular echo brightness, 239f
Pressure half time (PHT), 98f
Primary graft failure, 286, 288f, 289f
Pulmonary annulus, 20f
Pulmonary artery (PA), 20f
  banding, 53, 69f, 108f, 141, 146f, 169, 170f
Pulmonary atresia, 38, 40f, 107f
  functional, 88f
  with intact ventricular septum, 158, 159f–160f
  with ventricular septal defect, 121, 127,
    128f–129f
Pulmonary hypertension 269, 269f–274f
  estimation of diastolic pulmonary artery pressure,
    25f, 272f
  estimation of systolic pulmonary artery pressure,
    24f, 271f
  persistent pulmonary hypertension of the
    newborn (PPHN), 176f–177f, 273f
  pulmonary artery flow, 273f
Pulmonary regurgitation, 25f, 104, 109f–110f,
  121, 126f–127f, 130f, 233f, 269, 272f
Pulmonary stenosis
  valvar, 104, 104f–107f
  subvalvar, 101, 102f–103f
  supravalvar, 104, 107f–108f

Pulmonary valve disease, 104, 104f–110f
Pulmonary vein stenosis, 199, 206f–207f
Pulmonary venous anomalies
  cor triatriatum sinister, 199, 205f–206f
  partial anomalous pulmonary venous connection
    (PAPVC), 199, 204f–205f
  pulmonary vein stenosis, 199, 206f–207f
  total anomalous pulmonary venous connection
    (TAPVC), 199, 200f–204f
Pulsed-wave Doppler, 23, 23f–25f

R

Raphe, 92f, 95f–96f
Restrictive cardiomyopathy (RCM), 225,
  232f–236f, 256, 259, 260f, 262t
Rhabdomyoma, 263, 264f–266f
Rheumatic fever 241–245
  acute rheumatic carditis, 241, 241f
  rheumatic heart disease, 241, 242f–245f
Right aortic arch
  with aberrant left subclavian artery, 191, 192f,
    196f
  with mirror image branching, 191, 192f,
    197f
Right atrial appendage, 15f, 30f
Right coronary artery (RCA), 20f, 160f,
  215f–216f, 237f–239f
Right pulmonary artery, 16f, 19f–20f
Right ventricule (RV)
  function, 21f–22f, 270f
  hypertrophy, 121, 122f, 159f, 185f, 269,
    269f–270f, 274f
  morphological, 27, 32–33, 34f, 38, 141,
    141f–146f
Right ventricular fractional area change (RV
  FAC), 21f
RV FAC. *See* Right ventricular fractional area
  change (RV FAC)

S

Sano shunt, 169, 170f
Saw-tooth pattern, 181, 184f
Segmental approach to congenital heart disease,
  27, 28f–41f
  atrial morphology and situs, 29–31,
    30f–32f
  cardiac position, 28, 28f–29f
  type and mode of atrio-ventricular connection,
    33–36, 33f–37f
  ventricular morphology and looping, 32–33
  ventriculo-arterial connection and relationship
    between great arteries, 38, 38f–41f

Senning procedure, 146f

Septal bounce (constrictive pericarditis), 259f, 260f, 262t

Septal leaflet of the tricuspid valve, 53, 54f—56f, 81, 82f—83f, 85f, 87f, 141f, 143f—144f, 156f

Shunt (modified Blalock — Taussig, Sano), 129f, 169, 170f

Side-by-side great arteries, 41f, 111, 116f

Single outlet ventricle, 38, 40f, 147

Sinotubular junction, 20f, 99f—100f, 275f—276f

Sinus venosus inferior defect, 45, 46f, 51f

Sinus venosus superior defect, 45, 46f, 51f

Situs view, 4f 31f, 32f, 200f, 209f

Spectral doppler imaging, 23, 23f—25f

Stent, 126f, 127, 178f, 186f

Subaortic membrane, 89, 90f

Subarterial VSD, 53, 59f, 111, 112f, 116f—117f, 124f

Subcostal views, 4, 4f—9f

Subvalvar aortic stenosis, 89, 90f—91f, 188, 189f

Subvalvar pulmonary stenosis, 101, 102f—103f

Superior vena cava (SVC), 7f, 18f—19f, 51f, 171f, 203f—205f, 207, 207f—208f, 288f

Suprasternal notch views, 17, 17f—19f

Supravalvar aortic stenosis, 99, 99f—100f, 275f—276f

Supravalvar mitral membrane, 71, 74f

Supravalvar pulmonary stenosis, 104, 107f—108f

Swiss cheese interventricular septum, 53, 61f

Systemic venous anomalies
interruption of the inferior vena cava, 207, 209f
left superior vena cava (LSVC), 207, 207f—208f
levoatrial cardinal vein, 207, 207f—208f

Systolic anterior motion of anterior mitral valve leaflet, 89, 91f, 228, 230f—231f

Systolic pulmonary artery pressure, 24f, 271f

T

Tamponade, 253, 256, 257f—258f, 262t

TAPSE. *See* Tricuspid annular plane systolic excursion (TAPSE)

TAPVC. *See* Total anomalous pulmonary venous connection (TAPVC)

TCPC. *See* Total cavo-pulmonary connection (TCPC)

Tetralogy of Fallot, 102f, 106f—107f, 113f, 115f, 119f, 121, 122f—127f
with absent pulmonary valve, 109f, 121, 130f—131f
with pulmonary atresia, 121, 127, 128f—129f

TGA. *See* Transposition of the great arteries (TGA)

Tissue doppler imaging, 26, 26f, 227f, 233f, 235f, 261f

Total anomalous pulmonary venous connection (TAPVC), 199, 200f—204f
cardiac, 200f, 202f—203f
infracardiac, 200f—202f
mixed type, 200f, 204f
supracardiac, 200f, 203f—204f

Total cavo-pulmonary connection (TCPC), 169, 171f—172f

Transitional AVSD, 63, 64f, 66f—67f

Transposition of the great arteries (TGA), 133, 133f—139f
with pulmonary stenosis, 134f—136f
with ventricular septal defect, 134f—136f

Tricuspid annular plane systolic excursion (TAPSE), 22f, 270f

Tricuspid annulus, 19f

Tricuspid atresia, 35f, 81, 155, 162, 162f—165f

Tricuspid regurgitation, 24f—25f, 81, 83f—87f, 138f, 143f—144f, 156f, 159f, 233f, 245f, 249f, 271f—272f

Tricuspid stenosis, 83f

Tricuspid valve, 81, 82f—88f, 162, 162f—165f, 245f, 270f
atresia, 35f, 81, 155, 162, 162f—165f
dysplasia, 81, 82f,
ebsteinoid malformation, 141, 143f
fenestrated, 81f, 87f
overriding and/or straddling, 36, 37f, 81, 82f, 166f
prolapse, 82f

Trifoliate left AV valve, 63, 64f

Trisomy 21, 63, 280

Truncal valve dysplasia, 147, 151f

Truncus arteriosus, 38, 40f, 147, 148f—154f

Tuberous sclerosis, 103f, 263, 264f—265f

Tumors (cardiac). *See* Cardiac tumors

Turner syndrome, 279, 279f

U

Unbalanced atrio-ventricular septal defect, 65f, 66f, 155, 161, 161f

Unroofed coronary sinus 52f

V

Vascular rings
double aortic arch, 191, 192f—195f
Kommerell diverticulum, 192f, 196f

Vascular rings (*Continued*)
left aortic arch with aberrant right subclavian artery, 191, 197f
left pulmonary artery sling, 191, 192f, 198f
right aortic arch with aberrant left subclavian artery, 191, 192f, 196f
right aortic arch with mirror image branching, 191, 192f, 197f
Vegetation, 247f–251f
Ventricular interdependance, 256f
Ventricular morphology and looping, 32–33
Ventricular septal defects (VSDs), 53, 54f–62f
apical, 61f
doubly committed, 53, 59f, 111, 112f, 116f–117f, 124f
inlet, 53, 63, 64f–65f, 82f, 118f, 144f, 161f
malalignment, 53, 58f, 91f, 121, 188
multiple, 53, 61f, 155
muscular, 53, 54f, 57f, 60f–61f
patch closure, 62f, 70f, 119f, 126f
perimembranous, 53, 54f–57f, 97f, 102f, 273f
subaortic, 111, 112f–113f, 115f, 124f
subarterial, 53, 59f, 111, 112f, 116f–117f, 124f
subpulmonary, 116f
Ventriculo-arterial connection and relationship between great arteries, 38, 38f–41f
Ventriculo-arterial discordance, 41f, 133, 134f–139f, 141, 141f–146f
Ventriculo-arterial junction, 27, 161
VSDs. *See* Ventricular septal defects (VSDs)

W

Whale tale sign, 203f
Williams syndrome, 99f, 100f, 275, 275f–276f
Wilms tumor, 268f

Z

Zone of apposition, 63, 67f–70f

Printed and bound by CPI Group (UK) Ltd, Croydon, CR0 4YY

03/10/2024

01040373-0003